Psychological aspects of myocardial infarction and coronary care

Psychological aspects of myocardial infarction and coronary care

Edited by

W. DOYLE GENTRY, Ph.D.

Associate Professor and Head, Division of
Medical Psychology, Department of Psychiatry,
University of Texas Medical Branch at
Galveston, Galveston, Texas

REDFORD B. WILLIAMS, Jr., M.D.

Professor of Psychiatry, Assistant Professor of Medicine,
Duke University Medical Center,
Durham, North Carolina

SECOND EDITION

The C. V. Mosby Company

ST. LOUIS • TORONTO • LONDON 1979

SECOND EDITION

Printed in the United States of America

The C. V. Mosby Company
11830 Westline Industrial Drive, St. Louis, Missouri 63141

Library of Congress Cataloging in Publication Data

Gentry, William Doyle, 1943-
Psychological aspects of myocardial infarction and coronary care.

Includes bibliographies and index.
1. Heart—Infarction—Psychological aspects.
2. Coronary heart disease—Psychological aspects.
3. Coronary care units. I. Williams, Redford Brown, 1940- II. Title. [DNLM: 1. Coronary care units. 2. Coronary disease—Psychology. WG300.3 P974 (P)]
RC685.I6G4 1979 616.1'2 79-2554
ISBN 0-8016-1796-0

VT/M/M 9 8 7 6 5 4 3 2 1 03/A/345

Contributors

Ned H. Cassem, M.D.

Harvard Medical School at Massachusetts General Hospital, Boston, Massachusetts

Kathleen Dracup, R.N., M.N.

School of Nursing, University of California at Los Angeles, Los Angeles, California

Thomas F. Garrity, Ph.D.

University of Kentucky College of Medicine, Lexington, Kentucky

W. Doyle Gentry, Ph.D.

University of Texas Medical Branch at Galveston, Galveston, Texas

A. Dale Gulledge, M.D.

The Cleveland Clinic, Cleveland, Ohio

Thomas P. Hackett, M.D.

Harvard Medical School at Massachusetts General Hospital, Boston, Massachusetts

C. David Jenkins, Ph.D.

Boston University School of Medicine, Boston, Massachusetts

James J. Lynch, Ph.D.

University of Maryland School of Medicine, Baltimore, Maryland

Martin B. Marx, Ph.D.

University of Kentucky College of Medicine, Lexington, Kentucky

D. Kenneth Mitchell, Ph.D.

University of North Carolina School of Medicine, Chapel Hill, North Carolina

Kristine Nelson, R.N., M.S.N.

Harvard Medical School at Massachusetts General Hospital, Boston, Massachusetts

Carole Schornagel Orleans, Ph.D.

Duke University Medical Center, Durham, North Carolina

R. R. Rich, R.N., M.S.N.

Harvard Medical School of Massachusetts General Hospital, Boston, Massachusetts

Sue Ann Thomas, R.N., M.A.

University of Maryland School of Nursing, Baltimore, Maryland

Cynthia C. Scalzi, R.N., M.N.

School of Nursing, University of California at Los Angeles, Los Angeles, California

Redford B. Williams, Jr., M.D.

Duke University Medical Center, Durham, North Carolina

To

the readers of the first edition

whose feedback served to encourage us in our efforts at continuing education

Preface

In 1975, we edited *Psychological Aspects of Myocardial Infarction and Coronary Care* in response to our increasing concern that care-givers typically involved in diagnosing and treating patients with myocardial infarction were collectively uninformed about the available literature on the psychological aspects of coronary disease and coronary care. This first edition was also an attempt to bring together under one cover a broad range of relevant information on this topic that had previously been offered in a rather specialized, fragmented manner in a large number of psychological, psychiatric, and medical publications.

The general response to the first edition was extremely positive. This fact is attested to by the large number of letters we received from care-givers working in cardiology who read the text, the impressive number of sales both domestic and foreign, the favorable reviews of the text in various nursing and medical journals around the world, and also from the generous comments of readers at scientific and professional meetings we attended during the past 4 years. Our primary goal in editing the text was in fact realized, namely a large number of professionals actually using the book in their day-to-day dealings with cardiac patients.

This positive response to the first edition has stimulated us to edit a second edition of this text, which hopefully will serve as part of the continuing education of care-givers working with myocardial infarction and other types of coronary patients. With this purpose in mind, we have chosen not to simply update the material in the first edition; rather, we have made changes in the material presented that reflects shifts in emphasis and new knowledge in the field since 1975. Five of the original chapters were retained and updated; six additional chapters were invited to further extend our thinking and clinical expertise in areas such as intervention and cardiac rehabilitation. Thus, the second edition does not supplant the first edition; on the contrary, the second edition represents an entirely new and supplementary text that should be read in conjunction with the first edition for the most complete appreciation of what is currently known in this area of clinical medicine and also what types of advances we have made in our basic understanding of diagnostic and therapeutic issues for myocardial infarction patients during the past 5 years.

As with the first edition, we felt that the best view of the psychological aspects of coronary disease would come from inviting chapters from those persons most familiar with the subject matter, rather than trying to write the whole book ourselves. As before, we also invited material from a variety of professionals working in this field—nurses, cardiologists, psychologists, psychiatrists, and sociologists. The positive feedback concerning the first edition had shown that this format was a key element in making the book useful to those persons working with coronary patients. Again, we tried to include original writings by clinicians and researchers from a variety of well-known universities and medical centers.

As with the first edition, we arranged the chapters to reflect the continuum of relationships between psychological variables and coronary disease including issues of etiology, acute care behavior, cardiac rehabilitation, and intervention. In the second edition, we have tried to present a more balanced view of these relationships, giving more individual treatment and emphasis to issues of rehabilitation and intervention. This, we believe, reflects the shift in emphasis and research findings that has come about since 1975.

As always, we are thankful to the contributors who took time from their busy schedules to either update their chapters or to write the newly invited chapters. Without their willingness to provide this material, there would be no second edition. Their continuing enthusiasm and commitment to the educational effort of which this book plays a part has been most appreciated. As before, our task as editors was made both easy and enjoyable.

In addition, we wish to acknowledge the support and encouragement of the Departments of Medicine and Psychiatry at Duke University Medical Center and to the many cardiac patients with whom we have continued to interact both as researchers and as clinicians.

W. Doyle Gentry
Redford B. Williams, Jr.

Contents

Introduction, 1

Section one **Etiology**

1 The coronary-prone personality, 5
C. David Jenkins

2 Critical life events and coronary disease, 31
Thomas F. Garrity and Martin B. Marx

3 Physiological mechanisms underlying the association between psychosocial factors and coronary disease, 50
Redford B. Williams, Jr.

Section two **Acute care**

4 Preadmission behavior, 67
W. Doyle Gentry

5 Human contact, coping, and cardiac function in coronary patients, 78
Sue Ann Thomas and James J. Lynch

6 The nurse in the coronary care unit, 90
Ned H. Cassem, Kristine Nelson, and R. R. Rich

Section three **Rehabilitation**

7 Psychological aftermaths of myocardial infarction, 113
A. Dale Gulledge

8 Vocational rehabilitation and the coronary patient, 131
D. Kenneth Mitchell

Section four Intervention

9 Psychological intervention in myocardial infarction, 149
Thomas P. Hackett and Ned H. Cassem

10 Sexual counseling of cardiac patients, 162
Cynthia C. Scalzi and Kathleen Dracup

11 Behavioral approaches to risk reduction in coronary patients, 172
Carole Schornagel Orleans

Psychological aspects of myocardial infarction and coronary care

Introduction

Coronary disease is the major cause of illness and death in the United States and in much of the industrialized world today. Massive research efforts now underway are aimed at reducing the toll of morbidity and mortality exacted by coronary disease; much of this research is directed toward identifying physical factors that increase the risk of myocardial infarction, with the hope that interventions to reduce such factors will reduce disability and death associated with coronary heart disease. It is striking that many of the known risk factors are intimately bound up with life-styles, leading to the realization that to reduce risk it is necessary to change behavior. In addition to involvement with the known physical risk factors, many physicians, nurses, and clinical researchers in the field of coronary disease are convinced that psychological factors are also directly implicated in determining myocardial infarction and its outcome.

This edition surveys what is currently known, as well as what we need to know but as yet do not, concerning the role of psychological factors in all phases of coronary disease, from etiology through rehabilitation. In contrast to the first edition, we have expanded the section dealing with intervention, so that physicians, nurses, and other health care providers might become better informed regarding the recently developed behavioral approaches to reducing the impact of psychological factors on coronary disease and its outcomes.

The first section, Etiology, highlights the growing evidence for the direct involvement of psychological factors in the pathogenesis of coronary disease. Jenkins, in Chapter 1, reviews the evidence linking the Type A or coronary-prone behavior pattern with increased risk of suffering clinical coronary disease events as well as with increased levels of coronary atherosclerosis. In Chapter 2, Garrity and Marx describe the possible roles played by critical life events in the development of coronary disease, thereby extending the focus from the individual to events in his environment. Finally, in Chapter 3, Williams considers the possible physiological mechanisms whereby the factors described in the first two chapters may be influencing the development of coronary disease.

The second section, Acute Care, deals with those psychological issues that arise in the setting of acute myocardial infarction just prior to and during the hospital phase of care. As Gentry notes in Chapter 4, some 50% to 70% of those patients who die suddenly from acute myocardial infarction do so within 1 hour after the onset of symptoms; therefore, it is most important for health care providers to be aware of those psychological factors that appear responsible for patient delay in seeking medical attention. In Chapter 5, Thomas and Lynch make a strong case for the need to reduce fragmentation among the various elements making up the acute care situation: the structure of the CCU, the personnel in the CCU, and the patient in the CCU. In Chapter 6, Cassem, Nelson, and Rich focus more closely on the nurse as a key member of the CCU team, drawing extensively on their own clinical experience to illustrate the principles they wish to communicate.

The third section, Rehabilitation, considers the wide gamut of psychological influences that can determine the patient's ultimate success in reassuming the well role following discharge from the hospital. In Chapter 7, Gulledge surveys the psychosocial factors that affect the patient's emotional and behavioral adjustment during the recovery and rehabilitation process. Return to work is one of the critical outcome parameters in coronary disease, and in Chapter 8, Mitchell reviews those psychological issues involved in this aspect of the rehabilitation process.

The use of psychological and behavioral knowledge and techniques to reduce the adverse effects of psychological influences on the course of coronary disease is the focus of the last section, Intervention. In Chapter 9, Hackett and Cassem summarize specific techniques to either prevent unnecessary problems and complications or to treat them once they become manifest at each phase of illness—preadmission, acute care, and recovery. Scalzi and Dracup, in Chapter 10, review the sexual problems that often arise during the recovery phase, along with specific means of dealing with these often unnecessary problems. In Chapter 11, Orleans surveys those behavioral techniques that have been found useful in reducing the presence of factors that place the individual at risk to develop coronary disease.

SECTION ONE

ETIOLOGY

1

The coronary-prone personality

C. DAVID JENKINS

ORIGINS OF THE CONCEPT OF THE CORONARY-PRONE BEHAVIOR PATTERN

The physicians of antiquity were astute observers of the human condition both in sickness and in health. The clinical descriptions of many disease syndromes, even rather infrequent ones, provided by these early physicians have in many instances remained unsurpassed even to the present day in their comprehensiveness and eloquence. Although clinical descriptions of angina pectoris date back about 200 years, the first comprehensive clinical description of myocardial infarction is considered by many to have first been offered in the twentieth century. Taken together, these observations suggest that coronary disease is indeed a relatively recent phenomenon in the history of the human species and that the modern epidemic of myocardial infarction is one of our civilization's newer products.

Almost from the time of its emergence as a common disease, observant clinicians noted that people with coronary disease, particularly its younger victims, were somehow different on the average from their unafflicted neighbors. Dr. John Hunter (1729-1793), afflicted with angina pectoris, once stated that his life was "in the hands of any rascal who chooses to annoy me." He died while attending a board meeting at St. George's Hospital. Sir William Osler wrote in 1897, "I believe that the high pressure at which men live and the habit of working the machine to its maximum capacity are responsible for (arterial degeneration) rather than excesses in eating and drinking. . . ."[9] Other early examples could be cited to support this basic hypothesis that emotions and behavior relate to the development of coronary disease. (A more complete historical exposition is given by Leibowitz.[44])

To Osler's description of the coronary patient striving for success in a responsible but high-pressured way, the Menningers[51] added the concept of strong aggressive tendencies that were usually strictly repressed. Kemple[40] combined these notions and added the assertion that coronary patients seemed to have limited introversive experiences, limited creative thought, a constriction of imagination, and a lack of sensitivity to subtle nuances within their environments.

Other clinicians and researchers offered additional suggestions as to personality and behavioral characteristics associated with a high risk of coronary disease, but many of these assertions have fallen from favor through lack of support from later empirical studies.

Perhaps the greatest progress toward an integrated description of the psychological and behavioral contribution to coronary disease has come from the work of Friedman[17] and Rosenman.[57] These cardiologists have for over 20 years pursued a series of laboratory, clinical, and epidemiological studies of the role of behavior and the central nervous system in the pathogenesis of coronary disease. Friedman defines the coronary-prone behavior pattern as "a characteristic action-emotion complex which is exhibited by those individuals who are engaged in a relatively *chronic struggle* to obtain an *unlimited* number of *poorly defined* things from their environment in the *shortest period of time* and, if necessary, against the opposing efforts of other things or persons in this same environment."[17] People who manifest this behavior pattern are called type A individuals, and those who have the opposite pattern of behavior, a relaxed, unhurried, mellow, satisfied style, are designated type B individuals. The following is a supplementary definition of the behavior pattern:

> The coronary-prone behavior pattern is considered to be an overt behavioral syndrome or style of living characterized by *extremes* of competitiveness, striving for achievement, aggressiveness (sometimes stringently repressed), haste, impatience, restlessness, hyperalertness, explosiveness of speech, tenseness of facial musculature, and feelings of being under the pressure of time and under the challenge of responsibility. Persons having this pattern are often so deeply committed to their vocation or profession that other aspects of their lives are relatively neglected. Not all aspects of this syndrome or pattern need be present for a person to be classified as possessing it. The pattern is neither a personality trait nor a standard reaction to a challenging situation, but rather the reaction of a characterologically predisposed person to a situation which challenges him. Different kinds of situations evoke maximal reaction from different persons.*

It is important to distinguish type A behavior from the concept of stress. The term "stress" has different meanings to different people; sometimes it is used to refer to a noxious stimulus or situation and at other times it refers to the reaction of alarm, discomfort, or pain in response to a noxious stimulus. In contrast, the coronary-prone behavior pattern is neither a stressor situation nor a distressed response. It is rather a *style* of overt behavior with which some people confront life situations, either pleasant or troubling, provided that some element of challenge is perceived to be present.

Numerous studies, both clinical and epidemiological, have shown that anxiety, depression, and neurotic defenses are associated with the risk of developing angina pectoris and perhaps also with the risk of myocardial infarction. These

*From Jenkins, C. D.: Psychologic and social precursors of coronary disease, N. Engl. J. Med. **284:** 244, 307, 1971.

studies are described at length in two review papers.[27,28] This probable contribution to the risk of coronary diseases, however, is quite independent of the risk conferred by the presence of the type A behavior pattern. In studies involving a variety of groups, measures of the coronary-prone behavior pattern have correlated inconsistently with measures of anxiety, depression, and neurosis. Caffrey correlated behavior type interview ratings (on a 5-point scale) with scores on the Sixteen Personality Factor Test.[10] Most of the scales had negligible correlations with type A rating and the largest of the correlations were in the .20 to .25 range. Zyzanski et al.[83] found clinically unimportant correlations between the type A score on the Jenkins Activity Survey and scales for hypochondriasis, hysteria, anxiety, and depression derived from the Minnesota Multiphasic Personality Inventory. Hiland,[25] however, working in a Veterans Administration hospital, found type A to correlate with anxiety scores as high as .37, and Dimsdale et al.,[14] working in a general hospital, found correlations of .25 to .30 with stressful life events and current tensions. Our conclusions from these findings are that while there may at times be modest correlations between type A intensity and the presence of anxiety, depression, and neurosis, the long-standing behavioral pattern and the disturbing emotional states contribute relatively independently to the development of coronary disease. This was shown quite clearly in one angiographic study that involved a variety of behavioral measures.[37]

EVIDENCE THAT BEHAVIOR PATTERN IS A RISK FACTOR FOR CORONARY DISEASE

Given the preceding definition of the coronary-prone type A behavior pattern, what is the evidence that this pattern is a valid risk factor for coronary disease?

The early clinical studies conducted at the Mt. Zion Hospital and Medical Center in San Francisco were criticized by some epidemiologists because they were based on small convenience samples and lacked strict research design. It is important to recognize, however, that the major thrust of these early findings has been supported and extended by subsequent large, rigorously conducted retrospective and prospective studies performed by different researchers in a variety of places. The Western Collaborative Group Study (WCGS) was the first large prospective study that included a measure of the coronary-prone pattern at intake.[60] A structured interview was developed that carefully observed the subject's vocal response styles and motor mannerisms as well as the content of his answers. Behavior type was rated on a 4-point scale: strong and mild type A and mild and strong type B. This interview procedure, despite its apparently subjective nature, has been shown to have high interrater reliability and strong test-retest reliability.[31] The WCGS was conducted as a "blind" prospective investigation in which the persons who rated behavior types had no knowledge of other coronary disease factors and did not participate in the subsequent diagnoses of the presence or absence of coronary disease. The responsibility for diagnostic outcome judgments was vested in a specialist in electrocardiography and a medical referee (cardiologist). Both of these physicians worked independently of the study and had no knowledge regarding the presence or absence of risk factors including behavior type.[60] Reports of the incidence of clinical coronary disease in previously healthy men after surveillance periods of 4½, 6½, and 8½ years have shown that men judged to possess the type A behavior pattern at intake incurred 1.7 to 4.5 times the rate of new coronary disease as men judged to possess the converse, relaxed, easy-going type B pattern. The relative risk ratio observed differed by age of the subjects and length of follow-up, with younger men, and shorter follow-up being associated with higher relative risks.[58,61,62] Subsequently, the results of a prospective study of coronary patients in Oklahoma by Bruhn et al.[9] show that type A behavior was strongly associated with risk of coronary death.

Similar findings associating type A behavior and coronary disease have emerged from retrospective studies of more than 3500 men as they entered the WCGS[60] and from the Trappist-Benedictine Monastery study of more than 1500 men in the United States and Canada.[11] Several case control studies have also used the structured interview and confirmed the importance of type A behavior as a coronary risk factor.[39,77]

Results of an autopsy study by Friedman et al.[19] revealed a greater degree of atherosclerosis in the coronary arteries of men judged to have been type A as compared with those rated type B. Improvements in the technology of in vivo estimation of coronary vessel obstruction have opened the way to the concurrent study of type A behavior and extent of atherosclerosis. To date, three studies have reported strong associations between interview ratings of type A behavior and severity of atherosclerosis as determined by coronary angiography. Consistent findings have emerged from double-blind studies by Blumenthal et al.[1] in North Carolina, Perosio et al.[55] in Argentina, and Frank et al.[16] in New York City. Results of the study by Frank et al. also showed the independent contribution of type A to risk after five other risk factors were controlled statistically.

Although retrospective studies are vulnerable to bias caused by the impact of disease on behavior, such an effect will probably be minimal or absent in the angiographic studies because all patients in both the high obstruction and the low obstruction groups were anticipating a common procedure (the cardiac catheterization) and neither they nor their interviewer knew how serious a condition would be revealed by the diagnostic procedure. Retrospective or prevalence studies are also influenced by selective survival, and the possibility that this may bias the result can only be ruled out through prospective studies.

Many studies of type A behavior have utilized a self-administered, computer-scored questionnaire for determination of the presence and intensity of the behavior pattern. This questionnaire, the Jenkins Activity Survey, was standardized and validated against clinical judgments of type A behavior done by the Mt. Zion investigators.[30,36] The test provides continuous scores on the type A dimension and on three of its major behavioral components as determined by factor analysis: speed and impatience, job involvement, and hard-driving conscientiousness.[81]

Results of eight studies to date have indicated an association between type A scores on the Jenkins Activity Survey and the presence of coronary disease. In the WCGS, 83 coronary patients under 60 years of age scored significantly higher than a sample of 524 men without coronary disease,[33] and in a study in Bridgeport, Connecticut, 48 hospitalized coronary patients (both men and women) scored significantly higher than 42 patients hospitalized for reasons not involving cardiovascular disease.[41] In both of these studies, the coronary patients exceeded the controls both on the type A and hard-driving scales. Three studies have been reported from Veterans Administration hospitals in the United States. Statistically higher mean type A scores were found in coronary patients than in patients hospitalized for other reasons at VA hospitals in Durham, North Carolina,[70] Houston,[22] and St. Petersburg.[25]

The Jenkins Activity Survey was also administered to a large population of American men of Japanese ancestry living in Hawaii.[12] Several years after administration of the Jenkins Activity Survey, a subgroup of men was identified who had developed clinical coronary disease either shortly before or shortly after taking the test. Although type A means were higher in this case group than in men without coronary disease, this difference became statistically significant only when either the presence of status incongruity or social mobility was taken into account. Those men possessing the type A pattern plus either of the social change variables had substantially higher risk than men with neither of these characteristics.

The Chicago Heart Association Screening in Industry Project administered the Jenkins Activity Survey as part of a total risk factor determination.[69] Among those screened were a substantial number of employed men with established histories of clinical coronary disease. In a multivariate analysis considering all major risk factors simultaneously, the Jenkins Activity Survey type A score was found significantly associated with the presence of coronary disease. The strength of this relationship was about the same as that observed for blood pressure and serum cholesterol.

The most recent replication of the ability of the Jenkins Activity Survey to distinguish groups with coronary disease comes from Inowroclaw, Poland.[82] The Jenkins Activity Survey was translated into Polish, back-translated to verify accuracy, and then the corrected translation was administered to groups of coronary patients, patients with rheumatic disease, and healthy employed men. The male coronary cases scored significantly higher than the healthy men on the type A and hard-driving scales. Men with rheumatic and arthritic diseases scored lower on the type A scale than the coronary cases but somewhat higher than the control groups. The Polish study is important in that it shows the cross-cultural validity of the conceptualization of the coronary-prone type A behavior pattern. It also shows that despite the attenuation of measurement that is inevitably associated with translation into a different language and a different social system, the Jenkins Activity Survey is nevertheless able to distinguish significantly between coronary cases and healthy persons and generates a similar pattern of scores as observed in studies in America.

The most severe test of a presumed "causal" association—and the approach least vulnerable to the influences of selection and bias—is a prospective study. There is now published evidence that the Jenkins Activity Survey type A score is also predictive of the risk of emergence of new coronary disease in previously healthy men.[32] In the WCGS, healthy men who scored in the top third of the type A score distribution incurred 1.7 times as much coronary disease in the succeeding 4 years as those who scored in the bottom third or type B portion of the distribution. Later analysis of the comparative strength of the structured interview and the Jenkins Activity Survey in prediction of coronary disease showed the structured interview to be a stronger predictor in this population.[5] There is apparently some additive effect of the two methods in that men judged type A both by the interview and the Jenkins Activity Survey had the highest rate of new coronary disease and those judged type B by both methods had the lowest rate.

While the combination of evidence from prevalence and incidence studies suggests that the coronary-prone type A behavior pattern may actually be involved in the etiology of coronary disease, this inference would be further strengthened if it could be shown that the risk of coronary incidence was proportional to the intensity of the type A behavior pattern (a dose-response relationship) or that persons who have a second myocardial infarction are more strongly type A than those who have only one infarction. The first of these relationships has already been shown for the Jenkins Activity Survey type A score and coronary disease.[32] The regression of incidence rate on type A score yields a linear, significantly positive slope, even though the relative risk of high scorers to low scorers is only 1.7 to 1. Among men surviving their first coronary episode, there is a stronger association between type A score and risk of recurrent myocardial infarction. Men who suffer two or more myocardial infarctions are 2.2 times as likely to have a score of +10 or greater on the Jenkins Activity Survey type A scale as they are to be found with a score of −10 or less.[34] The relationship between type A score and reinfarction in this study, as shown in Fig. 1, may be curvilinear rather than linear, but in any event is a continuous graded relationship.

Two studies of angiographic determination of atherosclerosis have used the Jenkins Activity Survey thus far. The first study, by Zyzanski et al.[83] at Boston University, showed a strong relationship of all four Jenkins Activity Survey scales

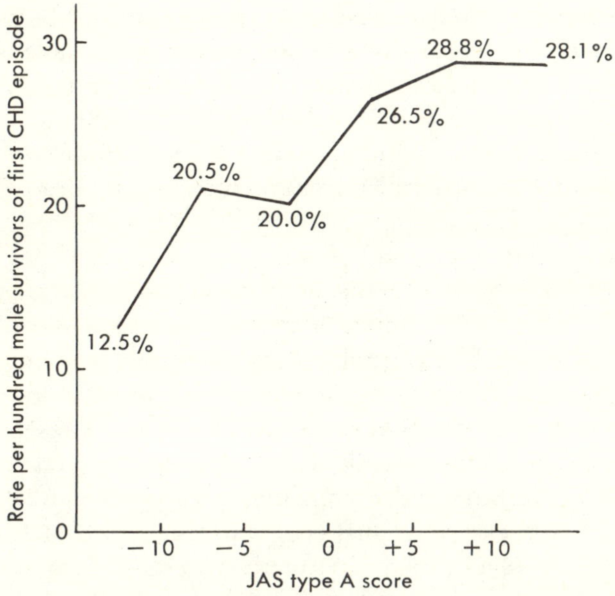

Fig. 1. Rate of recurrent myocardial infarction per hundred male survivors of first CHD episode (ages 39-59 years) arrayed by type A score.

to the severity of atherosclerosis. In a series of multivariate analyses that controlled for age, intensity of angina pain, and number of previous myocardial infarctions, the type A and factor H scores remained significantly higher in men with more severe arterial obstruction as judged by cineangiography. A study by Blumenthal et al.[1] conducted in North Carolina was mentioned before as showing a strong association between presence of extensive atherosclerosis and type A behavior as judged by the structured interview. This same study used the Jenkins Activity Survey but failed to find an association between its scores and extent of atherosclerosis. About half of the North Carolina sample was female and many persons, both male and female, were not engaged in wage or salary employment. Both of these considerations are likely to influence the validity by which the Jenkins Activity Survey measures type A for these kinds of persons. On balance, however, the entire array of studies relating the type A behavior pattern to clinical manifestations of coronary disease suggests that both the structured interview and the Jenkins Activity Survey are valid measures of the behavior pattern and that the type A pattern is a strong risk factor for coronary heart disease.

Clinical psychological considerations of the coronary-prone behavior pattern, as well as factor analyses of item pools designed to measure it, have suggested that the type A pattern has several independent features. Vocational involvement, striving for achievement, and excessive motor energy are among the components that have been identified repeatedly. Investigators in many nations have studied the relationship of one or more such components of the coronary-prone behavior pattern to coronary disease in one or both of its most common manifestations—angina pectoris or myocardial infarction. Most of these studies have been retrospective and have used groups drawn from medical institutions or large corporations.

Vocational dedication to the point of being a "work addict" has been found to be characteristic of coronary patients in locations as varied as Australia, the Netherlands, Sweden, and the United States. In Australia, Wynn[80] found coronary patients more likely than control patients to work many hours of overtime per week and also more likely to work at two or more jobs simultaneously. In separate studies in the United States, Bruhn et al.[9] and Russek[64] confirm the increased frequency of coronary patients who work at several jobs simultaneously. The excess of overtime work among men prior to myocardial infarction has been confirmed by Russek[64] and Thiel et al.[74] in the United States and Theorell and Rahe[71] in Sweden. MacKinnon[47] in Australia and Sales[65] in the United States present evidence that also implicates overload during the regular work shift as a risk factor. In the Netherlands, Van der Valk and Groen[75] found their coronary patients more dedicated to work in an exaggeration of the "success ethic" than were control subjects. Kits van Heijningen and Treurniet,[42] in a psychodynamic interpretation of these patients, call them work addicts, a description that is consistent with the findings of Liljefors and Rahe[45] in their study of Swedish twins discordant for coronary disease.

More recently the case control study of Ganelina and Kraevskij[20] in the Soviet Union shows that three times as many coronary patients as control patients were classified in a group characterized by high ambition and acceleration of their rate of work. Van Dijl[76] in the Netherlands constructed scales by factor analyzing a pool of statements claimed by prior researchers to be descriptive of patients with coronary disease. The two scales measured overactivity and exaggerated job involvement. Patients with coronary disease scored higher than both of two control groups on these dimensions.

Two prospective studies have associated facets of the type A behavior pattern with increased coronary risks. Bonami and Rimé[2] found that feeling of high achievement and job involvement on a projective test were predictive of future myocardial infarction. A prospective study of Swedish twins by Floderus[15] found items reporting time pressures and excessive job responsibility to precede the development of angina pectoris.

Problems and conflicts regarding vocation have been cited as being particularly common in coronary patients by Kavanagh and Shephard,[38] Sales and House,[66] and Groen et al.,[24] and by Groen and Drory[23] in a retrospective autopsy study. Additional studies implicate the sudden emergence of frustration or conflict on the job as a possible triggering mechanism for myocardial infarction. (A more extensive list of these studies is presented by Jenkins.[27,28])

There is also much evidence that striving for achievement and competitiveness is associated with the risk of coronary disease. The excessive vocational dedication and career striving previously described is certainly one manifestation of this underlying drive. The prominence of ambition, high social ideals, activism, and strength of will in coronary patients finds independent support in the work of Ganelina and Kraevskij.[20]

The research literature reports contradictory findings on whether occupational achievement per se is a risk factor for coronary disease, but there is more consensus that striving for achievement, with or without success, is so related. Wolf notes that coronary-prone men "strive without joy," and it may be that coronary disease disproportionately affects those whose striving is frustrated and seemingly unrewarded.[79] The type A person is an unrelenting striver, and it may be that without reward, chronic life dissatisfaction sets in and ego defenses become more exaggerated and less effective, culminating in the psychic exhaustion and emotional drain that Wolf[79] and Bruhn et al.[7] describe as often prodromal to myocardial infarction and sudden death. We view these additional psychological risk factors for coronary disease not as competing explanations to the coronary-prone behavior pattern, but rather as scenes and acts of a psychobiological scenario in which the type A individual is the most natural leading actor.

Another frequently reported characteristic of coronary patients—and part of the larger formulation of type A behavior—is the speed, impatience, and restlessness they manifest in their speech and actions. The candidate for a myocardial infarction is described as unable to sit down and relax when there is no work, gives the "impression of being tense,"[46] is "unable to relax after a hard day,"[78] and is "active, on the go, and tending to speak, drive, work and eat more rapidly."[6] (This last description derives from the prospective study of Brozek et al.)

Additional support for the fast-moving, restless component of the type A pattern as a risk factor for coronary disease is given in both the studies of Mertens and Segers,[52] who found time pressures and seeking of greater responsibility as characteristic of coronary patients, and the work of Thiel et al.,[74] in which coronary patients were found to have more rapid movement and excess drive as compared with a control group. The prospective study of Floderus[15] also noted time pressures as a risk factor for coronary disease.

Hostility is a common feature of persons with strong type A tendencies. It is particularly likely to be expressed when the person is impeded in any way from reaching his goals or even when he is slowed down and prevented from getting places or doing things at his usual speed. Theorell and Rahe[72] found that coronary patients became more hostile when slowed down than did a matched control group. In a prospective study of 6579 Swedish construction workers, Theorell et al.[73] again found that persons who admitted to becoming very hostile when held up in lines had statistically higher risk of future infarction.

The studies of separate facets of the coronary-prone behavior pattern reviewed in the preceding paragraphs have been conducted by investigators with many different theoretical backgrounds and hypotheses. They have attempted to measure behavior and personality traits in a variety of ways and have conducted their research in different nations. But, despite all this diversity and occasional contradictory findings on particular points that we have not discussed here, there is a surprising convergence of results that, taken together, provide additional support for the premise that psychosocial factors contribute to coronary disease risk and that much of this psychosocial contribution comes under the general behavioral syndrome called type A.

CLINICAL RECOGNITION OF THE CORONARY-PRONE BEHAVIOR PATTERN

The coronary-prone behavior pattern (CPBP) is best assessed by observing the subject in action. This behavior pattern occurs in women as well as in men, but because coronary disease strikes men two to six times more often than women, depending on age, it has been studied much more thoroughly in men. Increased research attention to the coronary-prone behavior pattern in women has only recently been initiated. For these reasons, our descriptions of the type A pattern will be given in terms of the masculine gender for sake of simplicity of expression. The same clinical symptoms, however, also mark type A behavior in women.

Type A behavior manifests itself in values, style of thought, manner of interpersonal relationships, response patterns, gestures and movements, facial expressions, rhythm of breathing, and speed, volume, and modulation of speech. The type A individual will direct himself sharply toward his goals, will gesture with abrupt assertive movements, will speak rapidly with bursts of amplitude for emphasis, and, by posture and concentration, will show an intensity of involvement and a lack of openness to extraneous stimuli not related to his selected goals. The type B person is more relaxed and open to the environment. He may accomplish as much work in a given time as the type A, but his movements are more modulated, his voice is even and unhurried, and he does not appear to be as intensely involved. He is not bothered by small diversions from the immediate goal.

The coronary-prone behavior pattern probably originates from deep-seated foundations of the personality. However, it is judged strictly on the basis of overt behavior. This behavior is usually best seen when an individual is actively responding to things that are important to him or in some way challenge or frustrate him. This is why it is difficult, if not impossible, to ascertain the behavior type of a very sick patient or a person who is bored or has disengaged himself from interacting with his surroundings. Once a person is involved in an occupational task, a competitive game, an opportunity to show skill, or a frustrating situation that he wants to change or from which he wants to escape, a variety of behaviors are emitted that permit judgments about the individual's behavior type.

The following sections list a number of indicators of type A and type B persons. The categories and the items are neither mutually exclusive nor exhaustive, but they do give a broad picture of the characteristics of the two poles of the continuum of behavior that signals coronary-proneness.

Values

1. The type A person is conscientious and responsible in an intense, inflexible way. Type A's set high standards for themselves and are critical both of themselves and others when they fail to meet these self-established standards. In Reisman's terms, they are "inner directed" rather than "other directed."[56]

2. The type A individual prefers being respected for what he does, whereas the type B usually prefers to be loved for who he is. This leads to the type A having to maintain productivity to maintain his feelings of self-worth. Type A's feel ill at ease if they relax for too long a period and often arrange a shorter vacation to get back to doing "something useful." This is the "Protestant ethic" expressed with a vengeance. It is found in people irrespective of religious affiliation and derives from the need, common in type A persons, to continually prove one's competence and social worth.

3. The type A individual has more obvious cravings for recognition and power than the type B, but may deny this when asked directly. The work of Glass suggests that the "need to control" may be a cornerstone of the type A personality.[21] Those persons who have a calm, easy-going demeanor until confronted with the threat of some loss of some control over the things and people around them and who then overreact with hasty, demanding or aggressive behavior are clearly type A persons who managed a temporary type B veneer.

4. The type A individual is compulsively attracted to competition and challenges. He will often compete against himself when no one else is available, trying to better his own previous "record" either in quantity or speed. The type B person competes as a means of social interaction. He may also try to win but is not as upset by losing as is the type A. Type B individuals often engage in pastimes or sports just for the enjoyment of it and, unlike type A's, may not even keep track of how well they are doing.

5. The type A subject has few sources of gratification other than his job and competitive avocational pursuits and does not seek additional sources. The type B individual spends his time in a greater variety of pursuits and derives personal gratification from more varied sources such as family, friends, hobbies, artistic and cultural activities, or spectator sports. Either type A or type B individuals may

participate in civic, political, or community affairs, but type A is more likely than type B to be "a man of action" and to seek leadership roles.

Style of thought

1. The type A person pursues several unrelated lines of thought or action apparently simultaneously, for example, working while eating, calculating or planning while driving an automobile, reading while shaving, or "doing three things at once" while on the job.

2. The type A person anticipates what is coming next and begins reacting to it in advance. Psychologists call these acts "fractional anticipatory goal reactions." The type A has his key out long before he gets to the door, he anticipates what another person will do or say next, he starts answering a question before it has been completely asked. Type B's are not in this much of a hurry. They do one thing at a time, and while they are not usually sluggish, they don't often "jump the gun."

3. The type A individual appears vigilant in expression and posture. He looks alert and ready to move. The type B projects a more comfortable air. Type B's can relax more completely and for longer periods.

4. The type A subject is compulsive about getting things done, overcoming barriers quickly, and having his own way. In contrast, the type B places a greater value on sociability and hence is less abrasive in interactions with other people.

5. The type A person is competitive in his approach to everyday tasks. He battles the tasks at hand, whereas the type B approaches tasks with less overt needs for mastery. The type A fights the "time barrier." He sees all obstacles as challenges, pushes harder, and does not give up even when fatigued. The type B is more willing to accept inevitable delays and to "give up" when a problem cannot realistically be overcome.

6. The type A individual is a poor observer. He fails to register the details of his physical and social environment. As a result, he often is unable to recollect those parts of his experiences that were not at his self-selected focus of attention. One cardiologist, an art collector, typically asks his new patients whether they noticed any paintings in the waiting room. The type B patients can often describe one or more of these paintings, but the type A's may not even recall that any were present. Similarly, the type A lacks insight into his own style of behavior and into the effect he has on other people. Thus type A's often fail to note the extent of their own impatience or their irascible demands on others. Family members and work colleagues of the type A patient are often more perceptive informants as to his behavior than is the patient himself.

Interpersonal relationships

1. The type A person tends to be self-centered, whereas the type B person will usually show more interest in other people. A corollary of this is that the type A is

a poor listener. His spouse or co-worker may complain that he does not pay attention to what others say to him.

2. The type A individual cannot stay in the frame of reference of other people if it does not coincide with his personal interest or involve his work. This limitation follows from the egocentricity and narrow range of interest of the typical type A.

3. Feelings of anger are more easily aroused in type A than type B persons. Because many type A's rigidly enforce high standards of "good conduct" for themselves, they will struggle to inhibit expression of these hostile and aggressive reactions. A spouse or best friend can often give a vivid description of the anger and resentment a type A person experiences when delayed or blocked, yet the type A person himself will often deny the intensity of these feelings.

One cardiologist frequently interviews coronary patients and their wives jointly. He asks the patient, "If a car ahead of you is going too slowly and you are unable to pass, what do you do? Are you in a hurry to pass? Do you honk your horn? Do you curse at him? Do you mutter under your breath?" The patient often describes himself as waiting calmly for an opportunity to pass the slower car safely. However, the wife or other family member often reminds the patient that in fact he does honk the horn, curse, or otherwise become upset by having his pace slowed.

4. The type A person feels frustrated in his work situation more often than the type B. He is often upset by the demands of the boss and troubled that the boss does not know the difficulties of the circumstances under which he is working. The type A also usually feels impatient toward subordinates either for their slowness or the poor quality of their work. Type B employees often find themselves in similarly conflicted circumstances, but the intensity of their feelings of frustration is not as great.

5. The type A individual often expresses an overt bravado. He exudes a certainty of his own correctness, feels that his capacity is superior both to that of his bosses and subordinates, and believes that with effort he can overcome any obstacle. The type B is more likely to recognize his own limitations and fallibility. It would seem that in many instances the overt bravado of the type A really covers a deep-seated insecurity. In occasional situations of repeated defeat or emotional drain, the type A may lose his bravado and reveal the insecurity and feelings of inferiority that lie beneath the surface.

6. The type A person tends to be more aggressive sexually than the type B, but it is the chase that he loves most rather than the consummation. In hospital wards providing care for coronary patients after their transfer from coronary care units, the type A patient readily distinguishes himself from the occasional type B patient by teasing the nurses, telling jokes with sexual implications, and occasionally initiating physical contact.

7. In addition to the demands he makes on other people, the extreme type A

individual is victimized by his own behavior pattern. He usually has no insight into this tendency and overestimates the degree of flexibility he really has. People associated with the type A individual either are drawn in to become victims of his inflexibility or run the risk of incurring his impatience and resentment. The subservience of the type A person to his behavior pattern explains why he pushes himself beyond his limits, as through extreme competitiveness.

Style of response

1. The Type A person reacts rapidly. When participating in a conversation, the type A person begins his comments without delay as soon as the other person stops speaking. In fact, one of the marks of the type A person is that he will often begin his reply before the other person has completed his question or statement. This interrupting behavior, known as "speech hurrying," increases the tempo of conversation and makes the other participants feel hurried. The type A person speaks with clipped syllables. Verbal flow is staccato, alternating bursts of words with hesitation for thought.

2. The type A person speaks with an air of certainty and emphasis. He accents words with a burst of volume. In contrast, the type B person lets his speech flow more smoothly in amplitude and pace and, hence, may sound more equivocal in his tone at times. The speaker who "drones on" when talking of things of personal interest is almost never a type A.

Two recent studies have emphasized the strength of association of voice characteristics with overall behavior pattern rating based on the structured interview. Both studies used highly reliable systems for rating volume and speed of speech from tape-recorded interviews. Speed of speech, volume of voice, and sudden increases in amplitude (especially with explosive consonants) were the strongest predictors found by Schucker and Jacobs.[68] Vocal emphasis, speed of speaking, and lack of delay in answering were the strongest predictors in the study by Scherwitz et al.[67]

3. The type A subject usually wastes no words. He speaks directly to the point. Type B's will often use more qualifying phrases, more parenthetical comments, and may circle around the point before getting there.

4. A type A individual can slow down his speech or writing on request, but it makes him uncomfortable. It is easier for him to speed up than slow down, but the converse is true for type B's. This principle was incorporated as one item of a performance test battery for the type A personality developed by Bortner.[4] Subjects were asked to write a phrase at their usual speed, then the same phrase more slowly, and then were challenged to write it extremely slowly. Some type A's were unable to go extremely slowly, and those who did often commented on the difficulties they were having. Type B's did this task quite easily.

5. When listening to another speaker, the type A person often gives anticipa-

tory nods and "ahems" while listening. He also may give short explosive laughs to quickly signal the speaker that he appreciates the point being made. The type B will listen intently but without needing to communicate that he has received the various points of the message and without appearing to attempt to speed up the other speaker.

6. When patients or subjects are questioned about situations that characteristically frustrate or block them, type A and type B individuals will respond differently. The type A often relives the tension or anger that he experienced in the situation while he describes it. He sometimes uses gestures, an angry tone of voice, or facial expressions to act out his original response or how he feels he would react if confronted with the situation again. Type B individuals do not get that emotionally or physically involved in their recollection of such events.

Gestures and movements

1. The type A subject gestures with tense, energetic movements. Both extensor and flexor muscles tend to be contracted, giving such movements an abrupt quality. The type B gestures in a "looser" style, in which the gesture starts slowly and trails off. It is not as "clipped" as the type A's gestures.

2. The type A individual often clenches his hands or makes fists when tense. He may strike a table with his closed fist to emphasize a point. The type B is more likely to shrug his shoulders or make open-handed, relaxed gestures.

3. The type A individual shakes hands with a strong grip and an active movement. The "dead fish" handshake, when it occurs, is more likely to belong to a type B.

4. When sitting or standing at rest, the type A person is less likely than the type B to remain still. The type A will "motorize," tap his feet, drum his knuckles, fidget in a rhythmic manner, play with a pencil, or shake a leg or foot. These motor movements tend to be rapid, rhythmic, and repeated. They give the impression of an overflow of excess energy bubbling out of the body. They are evidence of restlessness and on occasion may suggest impatience. These movements are not the usual "nervous tic" and do not usually have the same quality as "nervous fidgeting." The latter has a more uneasy, rambling quality, whereas the type A movements are more repetitive and constant in their form and more assertive in their style.

Facial expressions

1. The type A person often flashes momentary tense smiles marked by a lateral pull of the mouth with a tight horizontal lip line. This "grimace" is almost a tic in the extreme type A individual. In contrast, the type B person takes the time to generate a full smile and, because of more relaxed facial muscles, has more curve to his mouth and fuller lips.

2. The type A individual uses his brief smiles to give emphasis to comments and to reveal impatience. The smile of the type B is a more spontaneous expression of open feeling.

3. The type A person sometimes tenses his jaw muscles or grits his teeth when emphasizing comments. This gives rise to clipped speech. The type B does not hit consonants with such clipped distinctness. Facial muscles and movements of the head are more relaxed.

Breathing

1. The type B person breathes with a regular rhythm that is not seriously disrupted when he engages in conversation. The type A has more frequent breaks in breathing rhythm, heaving sighs or taking occasional, very deep inspirations during conversation.

2. The type A person will frequently inhale more air than necessary while speaking. In the middle or at the end of a sentence, this air will be released as an expiratory sigh. This type of sighing is not readily noticed unless the observer is particularly keyed to look and listen for it. The prominence of irregular breathing and sighing was first noticed on tape-recorded interviews with type A individuals.

3. This pattern of irregular breathing and expiratory sighing suggests that the type A person may be acting as if he feels under pressure or in an emergency. Apparently the activity of the sympathetic nervous system in this respect is substantially different from that prevailing in type B's, whose breathing is more regular and in whom sighing is usually absent.

It will be noted that these seven categories of signs and symptoms of the type A behavior pattern relate primarily to observable features of the style of response. One must also take into account the content of statements made by the person. Specific kinds of content indicative of the coronary-prone behavior pattern include indications that one is "always on the go," is exceptionally competitive, has high ambitions, demands high achievement of oneself, has a past history of promotion and recognition, has a past history of leadership in competitive situations, is always prompt, is always in a hurry (even when it is not necessary), is impatient and cannot stand to wait, is deeply committed to job or profession to the neglect of other aspects of life, is serious and precise about performance in all settings. The presence of this "content" can be determined through standardized interviews,[60] checklists,[3] or questionnaires.[36]

It should be emphasized that *no* one type A individual manifests all the characteristics listed in these pages, and even a slow type B person will show a few. It has been shown that type A is not a unitary concept or single dimension statistically but that it comprises at least three independent factors that correlate with the total pattern but not with each other.[81] Whether or not a person is judged type A clinically depends on an intuitive summing of the number of characteristics possessed and their intensity. The reason for including these signs and symptoms at much length is the clinical experience of Rosenman and Friedman, conveyed in their collaborative work, and my own further experience in studying the coronary-prone behavior pattern both clinically and statistically.

There has been a surge of interest in trying to determine which specific elements of the type A pattern, from among the many discussed here, are most strongly associated with increased risk of coronary disease. The answer to this question would be of great value in intervention programs to reduce type A behavior. It would limit the scope of the task confronted by the behavior therapist and would enable concentration, both by patient and therapist, on those aspects of the type A syndrome that would pay the greatest benefits in risk reduction.

The first study attempting to analyze the infrastructure of the type A behavior pattern contrasted men with clinically unrecognized ("silent") myocardial infarctions with matched control groups.[26] This design reduced retrospective bias because neither the patients nor the interviewers were aware of the presence of coronary disease at the time of the interview. Six components of the type A pattern were identified and the infarction group scored higher than the combined control groups on all six components, but this reached statistical significance for only one component—past achievements. The total score based on summing the scores for all six components significantly distinguished between groups.

Mathews et al.[48] factor analyzed an item-by-item study of tape-recordings of behavior type interviews with healthy men in the WCGS, some of whom later developed coronary disease. Five factors were extracted, only two of which were significantly associated with the overall behavior type rating. These same two factors—competitive drive and impatience—were also the only factors significantly associated with coronary disease incidence. Several individual items reflecting expressed hostility were also predictive of coronary disease incidence. These findings have not as yet been replicated in another project.

Prevalence and incidence studies using the Jenkins Activity Survey have rather consistently shown that the type A scale is associated with the presence or future risk of coronary disease, whereas the factor scales, each representing an independent dimension within the type A syndrome, do not regularly exhibit significant associations with coronary disease. Although the hard-driving scale has been found elevated in several prevalence studies of coronary patients and control patients, it is not predictive of future infarction and not associated with recurrent myocardial infarction.

Taken together, this body of evidence suggests that it is the combination of personality and behavioral characteristics that comprises the total type A syndrome as clinically conceptualized by Friedman and Rosenman that has the strongest association with coronary disease risk rather than any specific, focused components thereof. Clearly, further work needs to be done on this issue. The variety of individual components of the type A pattern that have been found associated with coronary disease by different researchers in different countries[27,28] and not replicated in subsequent studies underscores the need for cross-validation of findings before they can be recommended as a basis for therapeutic interventions.

IMPLICATIONS FOR MEDICAL CARE OF TYPE A PATIENTS WITH CARDIOVASCULAR DISEASES

In addition to the many clues to clinical recognition of the coronary-prone behavior pattern, the type A patient shows additional signs and symptoms of the behavior pattern; these make his recognition easy but his medical care more difficult. As indicated before, it is extremely difficult to distinguish type A from type B patients when they are acutely ill. This is particularly true for most patients during their first few days on a coronary care unit. Once a patient "becomes himself" again, he also once again becomes a type A or a type B.

More often than the type B patient, the type A will express bravado or "gallows humor" when approached for venipuncture or other invasive procedures. The brave front evaporates quickly, however, and the type A will show more agitation or fear and avoid watching the procedure. He will complain more loudly than the usual type B patient.

Once the type A patient believes himself to be on the road to recovery, he is likely to want to return to his usual life activities prematurely. He may even want to initiate and receive business phone calls from the hospital, have material brought to him to work on, and otherwise seek to prove that "neither snow nor rain nor atrial fibrillation shall deter him from his appointed rounds." The male type A patient (more than his type B counterpart) may initiate sexually toned byplay with female staff. This may be either flirtatious, provocative, or consist of expressions that tend to emphasize his manliness.

The type A wants desperately to be "in control." When he is not in control or not fully informed about plans for his care, he feels weak, looked down upon, and very vulnerable. The type A person will often be excessively demanding. He is particularly unaccepting of delays and will often seek to have ward regulations eased in his behalf. The egocentricity of the type A individual makes it hard for him to accept being on an equal status with the other patients in the unit.

Hospital staff members have a narrow path to tread in seeking on the one hand not to completely frustrate the rigid and demanding type A patient and attempting on the other hand not to bend to his will to the extent that the smoothness of ward functioning is reduced. Some special attention to type A patients, however, is both reasonable and beneficial to them, particularly in view of the frequency of this behavior pattern, especially among younger coronary patients.

Physicians and nurses can divert some of this type A energy toward therapeutic goals by enlisting the patient as a partner and ally in the recovery process. This means openly communicating the treatment plan and taking time to explain its reasons. Staff members should also be frank in explaining the type A behavior pattern to the patient who is in its grip, pointing out that retaining the pattern is part of his health problem and not part of its solution. Once this is understood and accepted, it may be possible to help the patient to change his behavior by leading him to perceive the more extreme elements of his type A behavior as ego alien, that is, as being something outside his true self. A therapeutic alliance thus becomes possible, with medical staff and the patient cooperating to avoid yielding to those strident inner urgings to be swept into type A activities.

There is evidence to suggest that type A behavior is an even stronger risk factor for recurrent myocardial infarction than it is for the initial episode, a characteristic not shared by many standard coronary disease risk factors.[34] There is no evidence at the time of this writing regarding the difficulty of changing the type A pattern or whether changing it in patients with coronary disease will reduce the risk of recurrent infarction. If such a relationship exists, intervention against the type A pattern is an important aspect of the hospital treatment of coronary disease. Even if no such relationship exists, the therapeutic alliance against type A, if successful, should make such patients more cooperative and easier to treat both in the hospital and thereafter. This is a legitimate goal in itself. (A further discussion of this issue is presented in Jenkins.[29])

Dealing with the root causes of the type A pattern may be the best way of reducing the intensity of its many forms of expression. A major goal is to shift the basis of a patient's judgment of self-worth from "doing" to "being." The patient should be encouraged and helped to value his own inner qualities and resources rather than to base his judgment of his worth on how much work he can do and how much he can achieve each day. Another goal is to increase the emphasis on the value of personal relationships and the quality of life rather than emphasizing "counting things." There should be a deemphasis on concern with time and on being "in control." In setting therapeutic goals the medical staff should avoid open-ended objectives; it is better to develop conservative goals and express them in specific terms. Staff should not reward overachievement lest they reawaken type A striving. Type A individuals are most likely to try to hasten the recovery process by engaging in more physical activity than is prescribed or by cramming a month of recovery progress into a week. It is obvious that this approach can jeopardize the recovery process.

While it is important to enlist the cooperation of family members and colleagues in the recovery process of every heart patient, it is essential to type A patients. Co-workers and family members, particularly spouses, can positively reinforce the patient for changing his behavior and his underlying value systems.

They can also alert him when he slips back into flagrant type A behavior, as when he deviates from the aftercare prescriptions either by overdoing them or underdoing them. The cooperation of close associates of the type A patient is particularly important because people with this behavior pattern have difficulty not only in controlling their style of behavior but also in observing it accurately.*

QUESTIONS ABOUT TYPE A BEHAVIOR PATTERN

Is the coronary-prone type A behavior pattern an all-or-none phenomenon?

Many discussions of type A imply that this is an all-or-none phenomenon, "either you have it or you don't." Actually, our descriptions of these two types represent the extremes of a bipolar continuum that is probably normally distributed in the population of the United States. In the WCGS the distribution of strong type A's (A_1), incompletely developed type A's (A_2), incompletely developed type B's (B_3), and strong type B's (B_4), was 10%, 40%, 40%, and 10%, respectively. Scores on the Jenkins Activity Survey were nearly normally distributed in the WCGS. In other populations the Jenkins Activity Survey scores may be skewed in one direction or another but have always been found to be continuously distributed within a single mode.

The Benedictine-Trappist monastery study[10] used an intermediate "uncertain" category in addition to the two intensities of type A and type B. A recent study in Belgium used the same system and also observed a symmetrical distribution across the five categories.[43] Friedman and Rosenman, in their most recent studies, have added this indeterminate category for individuals who exhibit an ambiguous mixture of type A and type B characteristics. We believe it is more effective, where possible, to characterize people by a score reflecting the quantitative balance of the type A and type B characteristics rather than to divide the entire population into a few major groups.

Is the coronary-prone behavior pattern merely a reflection of socioeconomic status?

Behavior type shows a modest correlation with occupational level; people in professional and managerial occupations have a higher frequency of type A behavior (and higher scores on the Jenkins Activity Survey) than people at intermediate and lower levels of the socioeconomic hierarchy of occupations. However, there are many type B's among top management and a sizable quota of type A's among the laboring classes. The reward systems of business and industry in most developed nations, however, tend to promote the rise of type A individuals to higher levels in the occupational hierarchy.[36,53,69]

Is the coronary-prone behavior pattern a risk factor for coronary disease among persons of all ages and in all population groups?

Most research on the coronary-prone behavior pattern has been limited to the subpopulations of industrialized societies most susceptible to coronary disease, that is, to men. Two limited studies suggest that type A women may also be subject to an increased risk of coronary disease (Rosenman and Friedman[59]; Kenigsberg et al.[41]). The ratio of type A risk

*A valuable series of specific approaches for changing type A to type B behaviors is presented in the recent book by Friedman and Rosenman,[18] particularly in Chapters 14 to 18. Interest is mounting in the use of counseling and behavior therapy to reduce the intensity of type A behavior.[13,63]

to type B risk of coronary disease is highest among younger persons and decreases with age. This situation is similar to that found to apply to such standard risk factors as serum cholesterol levels and cigarette smoking. There is no published evidence either for or against the hypothesis that type A is a risk factor after the age of 65 years.

Does the intensity of type A behavior reflect proportionately greater risk of coronary disease?

Data from the WCGS structured interview do not support the notion that the more blatant one's type A behavior, the higher the incurred risk of coronary disease. Men with strong (type A_1) or mild (type A_2) tendencies had high and equal risks of incurring coronary disease. Both type B groups (B_3 and B_4) had substantially lower risk, again without convincing evidence of a gradient.[61] This finding raises the possibility that a threshold phenomenon might be operating or that the cutoff points indicating relative intensity within type A or type B categories may not be optimally placed. In contrast to these findings, studies using the Jenkins Activity Survey type A scale have shown a "dose-response" relationship to the incidence of coronary disease, with high, middle, and low type A scores being associated with high, middle, and low incidence rates in the WCGS.[32] Intensity of type A behavior, as reflected by the Jenkins Activity Survey type A scale, is also related in a continuous fashion to greater risk of recurrent myocardial infarction in men already having coronary disease (see Fig. 1). The difference between these sets of findings suggests that the structured interview and the Jenkins Activity Survey may be sensitive to somewhat different facets of the type A behavior pattern or that the latter method may have better metric properties.

Is the coronary-prone behavior pattern predictive of different clinical subtypes of coronary disease?

Published reports show that both the type A interview and the Jenkins Activity Survey are predictive of future coronary disease, whether it presents clinically as acute myocardial infarction, silent myocardial infarction, or angina pectoris (without an infarction).[35,61] Many reports in the literature[49,50,54] assert that the psychosocial factors predictive of angina pectoris are different from those predictive of myocardial infarction. This is not inconsistent with recent findings that different subsets of items on the Jenkins Activity Survey are particularly associated with the later emergence of different clinical subtypes of coronary disease.[35] Future candidates for all three manifestations of coronary disease had different subsets of type A characteristics. Men who later developed angina pectoris were impatient and reactive in emotion and behavior to circumstances that blocked them. They acted out their type A behavior openly. Men who later developed acute myocardial infarction were serious, competitive, and concerned about time but reported much restraint in expressing these behaviors, particularly when it would make them socially conspicuous. Men who later incurred silent myocardial infarction endorsed a heterogeneous set of type A items not consistent with the two clusters just mentioned. There is evidence in studies in other nations that anxiety, neuroticism, and interpersonal conflict may be more predictive of angina pectoris than of myocardial infarction,[28] and similar specificities may exist for different aspects of the coronary-prone behavior pattern. This too is an issue needing further study.

How completely does the coronary-prone behavior pattern cover the psychosocial contribution to the risk of coronary disease?

A variety of sociological, psychological, and situational factors contribute to the prediction of the risk of coronary disease as well as to the prediction of the speed and adequacy of recovery from a variety of cardiovascular diseases. The coronary-prone behavior pattern is the most thoroughly studied of these psychosocial factors, and it makes a major contribution to the evaluation of both the risk of an initial episode of coronary disease and the possibility of recurrence and death resulting from coronary disease.[29]

While the coronary-prone behavior pattern is a major factor, it is by no means the only psychosocial factor; careful examination of other variables, preferably through prospective epidemiologic study, is greatly needed. Among the more promising categories of variables deserving intensive study are the sociological factors of social mobility and status incongruity and the psychological factors of anxiety, depression, somaticizing, and primitive coping efforts such as exaggerated denial and rigid, compulsive defenses. In addition, it may well be that the timing of the emergence of clinical cardiovascular disease is influenced by such situational determinants as life dissatisfactions, family conflicts, and life crisis. We have already speculated on the possible interrelationships of some of these factors with the coronary-prone behavior pattern, but these relationships need empirical documentation.[37]

SUMMARY

This chapter has traced the early observations and speculations regarding the role of behavior in the etiology of coronary disease. Recent research from many parts of the world repeatedly identifies a small number of behavioral characteristics as being peculiar to coronary patients. The coronary-prone behavior pattern as described by Friedman and Rosenman brings together many of these common themes. Much published evidence validates the association between the coronary-prone behavior pattern and its components and the risk of coronary disease, both retrospectively and prospectively. This behavior pattern is also associated with the risk of recurrent myocardial infarction in those who already suffer from coronary disease. It has also been repeatedly found associated with angiographic ratings of severity of atherosclerosis. Seven categories of indicators of the presence of the coronary-prone behavior pattern have been presented here to facilitate its clinical recognition both in healthy individuals and in patients being treated for heart disease. The implications of this type of behavior pattern for medical care in the hospital and later in the recovery process have been discussed, together with some strategies for attempting to modify the intensity of this behavior. Finally, a number of unanswered questions about psychosocial factors and coronary risk have been presented as challenges for future research.

The prevalence of the coronary-prone type A behavior pattern among cardiovascular disease patients and its importance in the course of heart disease and patient management make it essential that medical personnel understand its foundations in the personality, its reinforcements in our society, its manifestations in patients (and professionals), strategies for dealing with it in clinical settings, and approaches to modifying it as part of the longer term plan for rehabilitation.

REFERENCES

1. Blumenthal, J. A., Williams, R. B., Kong, Y., et al.: Type A behavior pattern and coronary atherosclerosis, Circulation **58:**634, 1978.
2. Bonami, M., and Rimé, B.: Approche exploratoire de la personnalité pré-coronarienne par analyse standardisée de données projectives thematiques, J. Psychosom. Res. **16:**103, 1972.
3. Bortner, R. W.: A short rating scale as a potential measure of pattern A behavior, J. Chronic Dis. **22:**87, 1969.
4. Bortner, R. W., and Rosenman, R. H.: The measurement of pattern A behavior, J. Chronic Dis. **20:**525, 1967.
5. Brand, R. J., et al.: Comparison of coronary heart disease prediction in the Western Collaborative Group Study using the structured interview and the Jenkins Activity Survey assessment of the coronary-prone type A behavior pattern. Presented at the Council on Epidemiology, American Heart Association, Orlando, Florida, March 13, 1978.
6. Brozek, J., Keys, A., and Blackburn, H.: Personality differences between potential coronary and noncoronary subjects, Ann. N.Y. Acad. Sci. **134:**1057, 1966.
7. Bruhn, J. G., McCrady, K. E., and du Plessis, A.: Evidence of "emotional drain" preceding death from myocardial infarction, Psychiatr. Dig. **29:**34, 1968.
8. Bruhn, J. G., et al.: Social aspects of coronary heart disease in a Pennsylvania German community, Soc. Sci. Med. **2:**201, 1968.
9. Bruhn, J. G., et al.: Psychological predictors of sudden death in myocardial infarction, J. Psychosom. Res. **18:**187, 1974.
10. Caffrey, B.: Behavior patterns and personality characteristics related to prevalence rates of coronary heart disease in American monks, J. Chronic Dis. **22:**93, 1969.
11. Caffrey, B.: A multivariate analysis of sociopsychological factors in monks with myocardial infarctions, Am. J. Public Health **60:**452, 1970.
12. Cohen, J. B.: Sociocultural change and behavior patterns in disease etiology: an epidemiologic study of coronary disease among Japanese Americans. Ph.D. dissertation in Epidemiology, School of Public Health, University of California at Berkeley, August, 1974.
13. Dembroski, T. M., editor: Proceedings of the Forum on Coronary-Prone Behavior. U.S. Department of Health, Education, and Welfare, Public Health Service, National Institutes of Health. DHEW publication No. 78-1451, 1978.
14. Dimsdale, J. E., et al.: Emotional correlates of type A behavior pattern, Psychosom. Med. In press.
15. Floderus, B.: Psychosocial factors in relation to coronary heart disease and associated risk factors, Nord. Hyg. Tidskr. Suppl. **6:**0000, 1974.
16. Frank, K. A., et al.: Type A behavior pattern and coronary angiographic findings, J.A.M.A. **240:**761-763, 1978.
17. Friedman, M.: Pathogenesis of coronary artery disease, New York, 1969, McGraw-Hill Book Co.
18. Friedman, M., and Rosenman, R. H.: Type A behavior and your heart, New York, 1974, Alfred A. Knopf, Inc.
19. Friedman, M., et al.: The relationship of behavior pattern A to the state of the coronary vasculature: a study of fifty-one autopsy subjects, Am. J. Med. **44:**525, 1968.
20. Ganelina, I. E., and Kraevskij, J. M.: Premorbid personality traits in patients with cardiac ischaemia, Cardiologia **2:**40, 1971.
21. Glass, D. C.: Behavior patterns, stress, and coronary disease, Hillsdale, N.J., 1977, L. Erlbaum.
22. Glass, D. C.: Stress, behavior patterns, and coronary disease, Am. Sci. **65:**177, 1977.
23. Groen, J. J., and Drory, S.: Influence of psychosocial factors on coronary heart disease: a comparison of autopsy findings with the results of a sociological questionnaire, Pathol. Microbiol. **30:**779, 1967.
24. Groen, J. J., Dreyfuss, F., and Guttman, L.: Epidemiological, nutritional and sociological

studies of atherosclerotic (coronary) heart disease among different ethnic groups in Israel: progress in biochemical pharmacology. In Miras, C. J., Howard, A. N., and Paoletta, R., editors: Recent advances in atherosclerosis, vol. 4, Basel, 1968, S. Karger AG.
25. Hiland, D. N.: Ph.D. Dissertation in Clinical and Community Psychology. Approved May 31st, 1978. University of South Florida, Tampa, Florida.
26. Jenkins, C. D.: Components of the coronary-prone behavior pattern: their relation to silent myocardial infarction and blood lipids, J. Chronic Dis. **19:**599, 1966.
27. Jenkins, C. D.: Psychologic and social precursors of coronary disease, N. Engl. J. Med. **284:**244, 307, 1971.
28. Jenkins, C. D.: Recent evidence supporting psychologic and social risk factors for coronary disease, N. Engl. J. Med. **294:**987, 1033, 1976.
29. Jenkins, C. D.: Behavioral risk factors in coronary artery disease, Ann. Rev. Med. **29:**543, 1978.
30. Jenkins, C. D., Rosenman, R. H., and Friedman, M.: Development of an objective psychological test for the determination of the coronary-prone behavior pattern in employed men, J. Chronic Dis. **20:**371, 1967.
31. Jenkins, C. D., Rosenman, R. H., and Friedman, M.: Replicability of rating the coronary-prone behavior pattern, Br. J. Prev. Soc. Med. **22:**16, 1968.
32. Jenkins, C. D., Rosenman, R. H., and Zyzanski, S. J.: Prediction of clinical coronary heart disease by a test for the coronary-prone behavior pattern, N. Engl. J. Med. **290:**1271, 1974.
33. Jenkins, C. D., Zyzanski, S. J., and Rosenman, R. H.: Progress toward validation of a computer-scored test for the type A coronary-prone behavior pattern, Psychosom. Med. **33:**193, 1971.
34. Jenkins, C. D., Zyzanski, S. J., and Rosenman, R. H.: Risk of new myocardial infarction in middle-aged men with manifest coronary heart disease, Circulation **53:**342, 1976.
35. Jenkins, C. D., Zyzanski, S. J., and Rosenman, R. H.: Coronary-prone behavior: one pattern or several? Psychosom. Med. **33:**193, 1978.
36. Jenkins, C. D., Zyzanski, S. J., and Rosenman, R. H.: Manual for the Jenkins Activity Survey, New York, 1978, Psychological Corporation.
37. Jenkins, C. D., et al.: Social insecurity and coronary-prone type A responses as identifiers of severe atherosclerosis, J. Consult. Clin. Psychol. **45:**1060, 1977.
38. Kavanagh, T., and Shephard, R. J.: The immediate antecedents of myocardial infarction in active men, Can. Med. Assoc. J. **109:**19, 1973.
39. Keith, R. A., Lown, B., and Stare, F. J.: Coronary heart disease and behavior patterns: an examination of method, Psychosom. Med. **27:**424, 1965. (See also Cassel, J. C.: Letter to the editor, Psychosom. Med. **28:**283, 1966.)
40. Kemple, C.: Rorschach method and psychosomatic diagnosis. Personality traits of patients with rheumatic disease, hypertensive cardiovascular disease, coronary occlusion and fractures, Psychosom. Med. **7:**85, 1945.
41. Kenigsberg, D., et al.: The coronary-prone behavior pattern in hospitalized patients with and without coronary heart disease, Psychosom. Med. **36:**344, 1974.
42. Kits van Heijningen, H., and Treurniet, N.: Psychodynamic factors in acute myocardial infarction, Int. J. Psychoanal. **47:**370, 1966.
43. Kittel, F., et al.: Two methods of assessing the type A coronary-prone behavior pattern in Belgium, J. Chronic Dis. **31:**147, 1978.
44. Leibowitz, J. O.: The history of coronary heart disease, Berkeley, 1970, University of California Press.
45. Liljefors, I., and Rahe, R. H.: An identical twin study of psychosocial factors and coronary heart disease in Sweden, Psychosom. Med. **32:**523, 1970.
46. Lovell, R. R. H., and Verghese, A.: Personality traits associated with different chest pains after myocardial infarction, Br. Med. J. **3:**327, 1967.
47. MacKinnon, A. U.: The psychopathology of ischaemic heart disease, J. R. Coll. Gen. Pract. **16:**253, 1968.
48. Mathews, K., et al.: Competitive drive, pattern A and coronary heart disease: a further analysis of some data from the Western Collaborative Group Study, J. Chronic Dis. **30:**489-498, 1977.
49. Medalie, J. H., et al.: Angina pectoris among 10,000 men: 5 year incidence and univariate analysis, Am. J. Med. **55:**583, 1973.
50. Medalie, J. H., et al.: Myocardial infarction

over a five-year period. I. Prevalence, incidence and mortality experience, J. Chronic Dis. **26:**63, 1973.

51. Menninger, K. A., and Menninger, W. C.: Psychoanalytic observations in cardiac disorders, Am. Heart J. **11:**10, 1936.
52. Mertens, C., and Segers, M. J.: L'influence des facteurs psychologiques dans la genèse des affections coronariennes. II. Données experimentales, Bull. Acad. R. Med. Belg. **11:**201, 1971.
53. Mettlin, C.: Occupational careers and the prevention of coronary-prone behavior, Soc. Sci. Med. **10:**367, 1976.
54. Ostfeld, A. M., et al.: A prospective study of the relationship between personality and coronary heart disease, J. Chronic Dis. **17:**265, 1964.
55. Perosio, A. M., et al.: Evolucion de la enfermedad coronaria cronica, La Prensa Medica Argentina **64:**27-32, 1977.
56. Riesman, D.: The lonely crowd, New Haven, Conn., 1961, Yale University Press.
57. Rosenman, R. H.: Emotional patterns in the development of cardiovascular disease, J. Am. Coll. Health Assoc. **12:**211, 1967.
58. Rosenman, R. H.: Assessing the risk associated with behavior patterns, J. Med. Assoc. Ga. **60:**31, 1971.
59. Rosenman, R. H., and Friedman, M.: Association of specific behavior pattern in women with blood and cardiovascular patterns, J.A.M.A. **24:**1173, 1961.
60. Rosenman, R. H., et al.: A predictive study of coronary heart disease: the Western Collaborative Group Study, J.A.M.A. **189:**15, 1964.
61. Rosenman, R. H., et al.: Coronary heart disease in the Western Collaborative Group Study: a follow-up experience of 4½ years, J. Chronic Dis. **23:**173, 1970.
62. Rosenman, R. H., et al.: Coronary heart disease in the Western Collaborative Group Study: final follow-up experience of 8½ years, J.A.M.A. **233:**872, 1975.
63. Roskies, E., et al.: Changing the coronary-prone (type A) behavior pattern in a nonclinical population. Manuscript from the Dept. of Psychology, University of Montreal, Montreal, Quebec, H3C 3J7.
64. Russek, H. I.: Role of emotional stress in the etiology of clinical coronary heart disease, Dis. Chest. **52:**1, 1967.
65. Sales, S. M.: Organizational role as a risk factor in coronary disease, Admin. Sci. Q. **14:**325, 1969.
66. Sales, S. M., and House, J.: Job dissatisfaction as a possible risk factor in coronary heart disease, J. Chronic Dis. **23:**861, 1971.
67. Scherwitz, L., Berton, B. S., and Leventhal, H.: Type A assessment and interaction in the behavior pattern interview, Psychosom. Med. **39:**4, 1977.
68. Schucker, M. A., and Jacobs, D. R.: Assessment of behavioral risk for coronary disease by voice characteristics, Psychosom. Med. **39:**4, 1977.
69. Shekelle, R. B., Schoenberger, J. A., and Stamler, J.: Correlates of the JAS type A behavior pattern score, J. Chronic Dis. **29:**381-394, 1976.
70. Stokols, J. J.: Life dissatisfaction as a risk factor in coronary heart disease, Ph.D. dissertation in Psychology, University of North Carolina at Chapel Hill, 1973.
71. Theorell, T., and Rahe, R. H.: Psychosocial factors and myocardial infarction. I. An inpatient study in Sweden, J. Psychosom. Res. **15:**25, 1971.
72. Theorell, T., and Rahe, R. H.: Behavior and life satisfactions characteristic of Swedish subjects with myocardial infarction, J. Chronic Dis. **25:**139, 1972.
73. Theorell, T., Lind, E., and Floderus, B.: The relationship of disturbing life changes and emotions to the early development of myocardial infarction and other serious illnesses, Int. J. Epidemiol. **4:**281, 1975.
74. Thiel, H. G., Parker, D., and Bruce, T. A.: Stress factors and the risk of myocardial infarction, J. Psychosom. Res. **17:**43, 1973.
75. Van der Valk, J. M., and Groen, J. J.: Personality structure and conflict situations in patients with myocardial infarction, J. Psychosom. Res. **11:**41, 1967.
76. van Dijl, H.: The A/B typology according to Friedman and Rosenman and an effort to test some of the characteristics by means of a psychological test, J. Psychosom. Res. **22:** 101, 1978.
77. Wardwell, W. I., and Bahnson, C. B.: Behavioral variables and myocardial infarction in the southeastern Connecticut heart study, J. Chronic Dis. **26:**447, 1973.
78. Wardwell, W. I., Hyman, M., and Bahnson, C. B.: Socio-environmental antecedents to

coronary heart disease in 87 white males, Soc. Sci. Med. **2:**165, 1968.

79. Wolf, S.: The end of the rope: the role of the brain in cardiac death, Can. Med. Assoc. J. **97:**1022, 1967.
80. Wynn, A.: The recognition of coronary proneness, Med. J. Aust. **1:**350, 1967.
81. Zyzanski, S. J., and Jenkins, C. D.: Basic dimensions within the coronary-prone behavior pattern, J. Chronic Dis. **22:**781, 1970.
82. Zyzanski, S. J., Wresniewski, K., and Jenkins, C. D.: Cross validation of the coronary-prone behavior pattern. Submitted for publication.
83. Zyzanski, S. J., et al.: Psychological correlates of coronary angiographic findings, Arch. Intern. Med. **136:**1234, 1976.

2

Critical life events and coronary disease

THOMAS F. GARRITY
MARTIN B. MARX

In western culture it has long been a belief, held by laymen and health practitioners alike, that certain events of everyday life may exercise a profound effect on a person's cardiovascular health. Coronary patients and their families often scan the patients' preillness lives in search of the events that caused the myocardial infarctions. It is part of conventional wisdom that pressures of work and worries about money and other family demands predispose individuals to heart disease. Occasionally, one hears of a sudden cardiac death that seems clearly linked with some shocking or provoking life experience. Individuals prone to angina pectoris may report a connection between emotion and onset of chest pain. Common as these perceptions are, the scientific validity of the link between life events and cardiac illness remains, for the most part, an empirical question.

In this chapter, we will review the evidence for and against the proposition that cardiac illness is influenced by life events. We will examine reports that seem to link single traumatic events with almost immediate cardiac death as well as studies that implicate the long-term accumulation of life changes as an instrumental antecedent of myocardial infarction, cardiac complications, and sudden death. We will also discuss the behavioral and physiological process whereby life events may be translated into negative cardiac outcomes.

SUDDEN CARDIAC DEATH FOLLOWING TRAUMATIC EVENTS

For decades, intriguing reports have appeared that suggest that emotionally significant life events may play a causative role in fatal cardiac malfunctions. Engel collected and analyzed 170 accounts of death after instances of extreme emotional arousal.[10] He reported that slightly more than half of these events involved the loss or threatened loss of friends and relatives. They tell of people such as the 61-year-old woman who collapsed immediately after receiving news of her sister's sudden death and died shortly thereafter of cardiac arrest. There is an account of an 88-year-old man without known heart disease who, on learning of the sudden death of his daughter, developed acute pulmonary congestion and died as his physician reached his house. Other reports in Engel's collection involved response to the threatened loss of a loved one. One of these is the account of a 40-year-old father who "slumped dead as he cushioned the head of his son lying injured in the street beside his motorcycle" and another of the 67-year-old woman who died "while waiting to hear news of friends in a disastrous nursing home fire."

Other types of loss events may also be pathogenic. Sudnow[55] presented a case report of sudden cardiac death following a marital breakup. A seriously ill man, hospitalized with a perforated duodenal ulcer and not expected to recover from his illness, made a remarkable recovery and returned home. On arriving home, he found that his wife had already arranged his funeral, disposed of his belongings, stopped wearing her wedding ring, and found a prospective replacement spouse. In great distress, the man began to drink heavily and soon returned to the hospital where he died of a heart attack. Loss of reputation or self-esteem appears instrumental in the emotional status of nine accounts reported by Engel; for example, the case of the "52-year-old college president who prided himself on his support of Black students (who) died when a group of Black students occupied the administration building." He also tells of the "57-year-old State legislator (who) died 48 hours after being convicted of bribery and sentenced to prison."

While sudden death after life events involving significant loss is apparent, fear-filled emotional arousal may be more common. Cannon's classic paper seems to fit this category.[6] He reviewed several anthropological accounts of "voodoo death" in which offenders of tribal taboos were cursed and subsequently died unaccountably. Cannon, a renowned physiologist, discounted the possibility that these deaths happened by chance and that they might have been caused by prior disease in the victims. It seemed more likely to him that the threat, supported by a strong social belief in voodoo, was so intense that fear, physical collapse, and death were the results. Cannon's accounts of "voodoo death" and those of others[64,67] generally described victims as becoming highly fearful and, subsequently, deeply depressed. Death usually occurred within several days, but occasionally after only a few hours. The proximate physical cause of death was thought to be a type of cardiovascular dysfunction.

Other accounts of fear-filled life events preceding sudden cardiac death appear in the literature. Engel listed several sources of fear associated with such deaths: fear of surgery,[2,9] experiencing upsetting anniversaries,[8,11] experiencing hospital ward rounds,[30] administration of last rites,[40] and altercation with another person.[23] He also reported that of his 170 accounts of death after emotional distress, no less than 27% were related to either "personal danger or threat of injury, real or symbolic." Engel gave accounts of the "63-year-old security guard (who) died after being bound by robbers" and the "45-year-old man (who) died as he stepped to the dais to give a speech at a testimonial dinner." His youngest cases were of a "3-year-old child who died when caught in a severe downpour and a terrified 4-year-old girl who died while having some milk teeth extracted."

Although sudden death after emotional excitation is most often associated with severe loss or fear of loss, there are reports of death following quite different types of events. Fitzhugh and Hamilton[12] described death after the excitement of viewing sporting events. Engel[10] found instances of deaths following positive life events involving effects of extreme pleasure, triumph, and relief. For example, there was the 60-year-old prisoner who "collapsed and died when he returned home to his family after serving a 15-year sentence" and the 55-year-old man and his 88-year-old father who died on meeting after a 20-year separation.

SUSPECTED MECHANISMS OF SUDDEN CARDIAC EVENTS

Let us assume for the present discussion that the instances of sudden death just described are, in fact, provoked by traumatic life events. We are left to consider two related questions: What physical malfunction caused these deaths and what specific physiological mechanisms explain the association between these life events and the physical malfunction causing death?

There is evidence that most of these sudden deaths involve heart dysfunction, most commonly a disturbance of cardiac rhythm.[10] The majority of sudden death victims are individuals with diseases of the heart and aorta.[10,33] Of those who die within minutes, "effective cardiac arrest, whether caused by ventricular asystole or by ventricular tachyarrhythmias" is most likely the cause of death.[10] Among deaths in males who die within an hour of illness onset, 91% may be attributed to coronary artery disease.[54] It is also clear that most instances of sudden death occur in later life when coronary disease is most frequently diagnosed. While Engel concedes that some of the deaths described in his 170 accounts are no doubt unrelated to cardiac malfunction, heart disease is clearly the primary culprit.

The mechanism linking psychological distress, physiological arousal, and negative cardiovascular outcomes is still very much open to conjecture. A familiar understanding of this mechanism was susggested by Cannon in his description of fight-or-flight defenses. In this view, man is innately capable of rapidly mobilizing stored chemical energy in the presence of some threat.[45,53] For example, when confronted suddenly by an attacking, angry dog, one experiences instantaneous increases of heart rate and blood pressure along with a myriad of other metabolic changes that support increased energy expenditures capable of facilitating counterattack (fight) or escape (flight) from the animal. In this case, man's unconscious reaction is to survey and appraise the situation; this is followed by an involuntary communication of the appropriate neural and hormonal signals to various bodily organs, which then subserve the needed behavioral responses.

In the healthy organism, this excitatory response is not only well tolerated, but is most useful in coping with acute challenges requiring responses of intense physical effort. However, when the heart or vascular system is weakened by disease, the fight-or-flight response can precipitate fatal changes.

This excitatory response involves arousal of the sympathetic nervous system and, as mentioned above, involves acceleration of heart rate and outpouring of a variety of stress hormones including catecholamines[32,37] and glucocorticoids.[20,38] The fast heart rhythms and irritability of the cardiac ventricles set up in this process are well documented[18,21,41] and may predispose to fatal changes in rhythm. In addition, the role of the catecholamines—epinephrine and norepinephrine—in coronary disturbances and sudden death have long been suspected.[31,43]

A study of a small number of patients hospitalized for heart attack helps to illustrate several of these points. Klein et al.[31] had come to expect an increase in patients' medical and emotional problems around the time of their transfer from the intensive coronary care unit to the general medical wards for further recuperation. Transfer occurred because the intensive care given in the cardiac unit was no longer needed as cardiac function stabilized during the first several days after the attack. However, patients often became anxious about the transfer, feeling that the move might place them in danger if further heart trouble were experienced. It was found that catecholamine levels increased as patients became upset around the time of transfer. (These hormones are produced in greater quantity whenever an individual experiences emotional distress.) It was also found that a variety of cardiac disturbances occurred in conjunction with these emotional and hormonal responses. In the case of seven transferred patients studied intensively, five experienced a rise in catecholamine excretion and each of these patients also exhibited some cardiac dysfunction ranging from minor rhythm disturbances to recurrent myocardial infarction and death. Subsequently, a program was implemented to prepare patients for transfer and to provide emotional support before, during, and after the move. In a series of seven prepared patients, only two developed increased catecholamine levels and none experienced cardiac complications.

While the excitatory mechanism just reviewed appears promising in explaining how traumatic life events may be related to sudden cardiac death, Engel[10] draws attention to an "inhibitory" mechanism that may also play such a role. While the excitatory response involves sympathetic arousal, the inhibitory response, characterized at the psychological level by "conservation-withdrawal" and giving up, involves parasympathetic dominance. The latter is manifested in slowing of heart rate. Just as fast heart rates may predispose individuals to arrhythmias, so also may slow rates lead to a variety of rhythm disturbances.[27,28] Engel recognized both of these neurogenic cardiovascular influences[10] and cited some evidence that rapid shifts in dominance between the excitatory and inhibitory phenomena may also lead to dangerous cardiac rhythm disturbances.[19] "In either event," he states, "these are ideal conditions for the development of cardiac arrest and lethal arrhythmias, especially in the presence of preexisting coronary disease."

CUMULATIVE LIFE EVENTS AND ILLNESS

Single, traumatic life events have already been seen to be possible causal antecedents of fatal changes in cardiac function. They serve to illustrate a theory that links a larger realm of life events with health status generally, in addition to cardiac status. The theory, simply stated, holds that when life events accumulate, especially changes requiring some degree of adaptation, individuals are likely to experience psychophysiological strain that predisposes them to a breakdown of health. In this section, we describe the origin of this psychosomatic theory and the accumulating evidence that life change is causally associated with illness. In the following section, evidence is reviewed that links accumulated recent life events with coronary disease per se.

The life events–health change theory is a subset of the psychosomatic theory linking functions of the mind with bodily illness. The works of Cannon,[4,5] Selye,[53] and Alexander,[1] early pioneers in this area of research, are antecedents of this more recent theory. In general, psychosomatic theories associate negative changes in bodily function with the psychophysiological struggle to meet and cope with a challenge, threat, or conflict. Normal, healthy adaptive responses can themselves cause illness when activation is prolonged, intensified, or otherwise deranged.

The early tendency in psychosomatic theory to link specific emotions[65] and personality configurations with specific illnesses has given way to the belief that psychophysiological disturbance results from an almost limitless variety of stressful stimuli leading to a large array of illness outcomes.[42] Prolonged psychophysiological arousal may therefore increase the susceptibility of an organism to illness and injury from infectious, chronic degenerative and emotional diseases. Hence, stress may be indirectly capable of lowering resistance to disease-producing micro-organisms and of setting into motion physical processes that can, in the long run, damage both the morphology and the physiology of organs and seriously tax the psychological coping capacities of the individual.

It was out of this perspective of psychosomatic theory that the life events–health change theory grew. In 1949, Holmes et al.[26] began to develop a method for measuring the amount and strength of recent life change experienced in individuals and for studying the effect of such change on health. It is Holmes' conviction that life changes, both desirable and undesirable, cause a break in the stability and equilibrium of life.[24] Thus, the adaptation process may place the

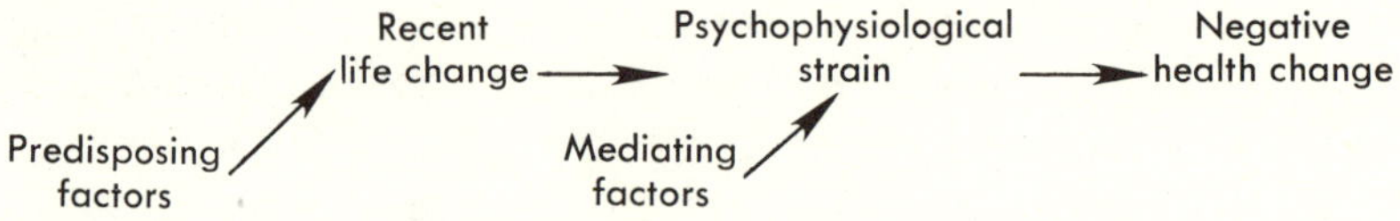

Fig. 2. Schematic representation of life change–health change paradigm.

individual under a psychophysiological strain that, in turn, is believed to increase the likelihood of a negative change in health.

Fig. 2 is a diagram of the model being discussed. The relationship between recent life events and negative health changes is mediated by psychophysiological strain. Simply put, life changes stress the person, causing the organism to struggle emotionally and physically to cope with the change; this struggle frequently results in a breakdown of health. Fig. 2 suggests two other elements for consideration in this theory. It is not unusual for some people with many recent life changes to remain healthy. At least part of the explanation for this resistance may be found in personal and environmental factors that increase the individual's coping resources. For example, a person with strong resources of love and respect may use these as a source of emotional and informational support for dealing with challenging life disruptions. Such resources, if effectively used, may prevent the person from experiencing psychophysiological strain and, consequently, the onset of illness. In a similar way, certain personality strengths could act to lessen the strain resulting from life change. Hence, a complete representation of the life events–health change model must include mediating factors capable of reducing the impact of events of health. Conversely, certain environmental and personal factors may potentiate the life change–health change relationship.

Fig. 2 also suggests the existence of factors that influence the occurrence of life change events themselves. Clearly, some of the changes that life brings are largely out of man's control, for example, a home destroyed in an earthquake or flood, the death of a friend, the closing of one's place of employment. Nonetheless, many life changes are controllable, such as starting a new job, marrying, moving to a new residence. It is possible that certain personal and environmental factors promote change-seeking behavior. Casual observation of friends and associates reveals that some seem most content in relatively quiet and unchanging life-styles, while others seek excitement, change, and a frenetic pace of life. Hence, no complete picture of the life events–health change model can exclude mention of the factors that predispose individuals to life change experience.

By 1967, Holmes and Rahe had developed an instrument useful in measuring recent life change experience.[25] Their Social Readjustment Rating Scale (Table 1) included 43 commonly reported life change events. Using a large panel of judges, they were able to determine and assign values or weights to each item in

Table 1. Social readjustment rating scale*

Rank	Life event	Mean value
1	Death of spouse	100
2	Divorce	73
3	Marital separation	65
4	Jail term	63
5	Death of close family member	63
6	Personal injury or illness	53
7	Marriage	50
8	Fired at work	47
9	Marital reconciliation	45
10	Retirement	45
11	Change in health of family member	44
12	Pregnancy	40
13	Sex difficulties	39
14	Gain of new family member	39
15	Business readjustment	39
16	Change in financial state	38
17	Death of close friend	37
18	Change to different line of work	36
19	Change in number of arguments with spouse	35
20	Mortgage over $10,000	31
21	Foreclosure of mortgage or loan	30
22	Change in responsibilities at work	29
23	Son or daughter leaving home	29
24	Trouble with in-laws	29
25	Outstanding personal achievement	28
26	Wife begin or stop work	26
27	Begin or end school	26
28	Change in living conditions	25
29	Revision of personal habits	24
30	Trouble with boss	23
31	Change in work hours or conditions	20
32	Change in residence	20
33	Change in schools	20
34	Change in recreation	19
35	Change in church activities	19
36	Change in social activities	18
37	Mortgage or loan less than $10,000	17
38	Change in sleeping habits	16
39	Change in number of family get-togethers	15
40	Change in eating habits	15
41	Vacation	13
42	Christmas	12
43	Minor violations of the law	11

*From Holmes, T. H., and Rahe, R. H.: J. Psychosom. Res. **11**:216, 1967.

proportion to the "relative degree of necessary readjustment" required by each event. The ratings by judges ranged from 100 for the readjustment required after the death of one's spouse to 11 for minor violations of the law. This approach to the measurement of life change has been criticized for not covering a sufficient range and variety of life change events, for assigning readjustment weights that only weakly approximate the individual responses of most research subjects, for including desirable as well as undesirable life changes, and for various other reasons.[44] Nevertheless, several studies of the rating scale have demonstrated that in various cultures around the world and with people of differing social and personal characteristics, the rankings of these various life changes were quite consistent.[27,39,66] Furthermore, the Social Readjustment Rating Scale has proven a reliable predictor of illness outcomes.

Results of an extensive group of studies undertaken by Rahe[46] has shown that the extent of life events experienced by young naval personnel in the 6 months prior to a 6-month cruise is predictive of their illness rates during sea duty. These findings inspire some confidence because of the use of a rigorous prospective study design that eliminates some biases possible in the less demanding retrospective design used in most earlier studies. Also, the use of a captive and confined shipboard population minimizes the effects of externally introduced sources of illness. Furthermore, the findings of Rahe in this American sample have been largely replicated in studies of Norwegian sailors.[49]

The relationship between recent life events and illness has been documented in a range of study populations and for a range of illness outcomes. In relatively young populations, illness outcomes have generally included minor illness, for example, upper respiratory infections and accidental injuries.[3,45] However, the review of Rabkin and Streuning[44] summarizes that "modest but statistically significant relationships have been found between mounting life change and the occurrence or onset of sudden cardiac death, myocardial infarction, accidents, athletic injuries, tuberculosis and the entire gamut of minor medical complaints." They also point out that psychiatric symptoms and disorders have been significantly predicted by life change scores.

While it is not the purpose of this presentation to comprehensively review the findings or the criticisms of this theoretical model, it should be understood that the theory is not without its critics. In addition to the criticisms of the Social Readjustment Rating Scale mentioned already, some have argued that the "statistically significant" correlations found in most of this research are clinically trivial. Some have wondered if even these associations are misleading and explainable without reference to the life events–health change theory. For example, it seems possible that the relationship could be caused by the tendency of some individuals to report many problems, be they of health or life in general. Such a propensity would build in a significant life events–health change correlation but would not support the psychosomatic links between the two.[17] It is also possible that the life events–health change relationship results from a correlation between the high life events score and the high utilization of health service regardless of the physical health status. In this case, the apparent life events–health change relationship would really be indicative of a relationship between life change and care-seeking behavior rather than diagnosed somatic disease. In spite of this type of conjecture, the weight of evidence continues to suggest a causal link between life change and health; but further research on a number of aspects of the model is needed.

CUMULATIVE LIFE EVENTS AND CORONARY HEART DISEASE

In 1971, studies began to appear that suggested that buildup of recent life events was predictive of subsequent cardiac pathology. In a pilot study of 39 Swedish victims of sudden cardiac death, Rahe and Lind[47] found that the intensity of recent life changes had increased over the last 6 months of the victims' lives as compared with the same 6-month periods of the previous 2 years. Information regarding life changes in the 3 years prior to death was obtained from a survivor of the deceased, usually the spouse. Previous work had shown that use of the spouse as a source of life events data compared well with reports of heart patients themselves.[56] The peak life change intensity was about three times the baseline level of life changes. This increasing of life change seemed to hold for victims both with and without histories of coronary disease. Studies of other illness have also shown buildups of recent life changes prior to the onset of illness.

Assessment of recent life change was, obviously, done after the cardiac event. We caution that an alternative explanation for the study findings may be that knowledge of the illness and death stimulates respondents to report greater life change events to help make sense of the cardiac event. Such selective recall would lend false credence to the life events–health change hypothesis. However, if this bias had been operating, it is hard to understand why the reporting pattern of increasing life change was apparent only for the 6 months immediately before the illness and not during the other periods prior to illness. While most of the studies reported in this section suffer the weakness of retrospective life assessment, one prospective study to be discussed below also demonstrates pre-illness life event buildup.[60]

A second source of bias possible in this sort of research is that premonitory symptoms of the cardiac event may cause a buildup of behavioral changes that are themselves recorded as life change events. In this case, life change is really a response to illness rather than a cause of it as postulated in the life events–health change model. In a study previously described,[47] this source of possible invalidity was handled in two ways. First, subjects with and without histories of coronary symptoms and disease were analyzed separately; the life change buildup was found in both groups. Second, the study eliminated from consideration any life changes reported for the year-quarter of death (quarter of the year in which death occurred). In this way, events caused by acute premonitory symptoms would not be counted as autonomous life changes.

Theorell and Rahe[59] reported on a study of survivors of myocardial infarction and a small group of healthy matched control subjects. As was the case with victims of sudden cardiac death, evidence was found of life events building up prior to the attack. While healthy control subjects exhibited no life change buildup, victims with no history of heart disease showed a buildup during the 2 years before the attack. Subjects with a positive history of coronary disease demonstrated a buildup that peaked in the second year before the attack. The latter peak tended to coincide with the experience of cardiac symptoms. Among these surviving patients, Theorell and Rahe were unable to find any relationship between intensity of life change and severity of the heart attack.

In a study of 30 myocardial infarction survivors with no history of coronary disease, Rahe and Paasikivi[48] found evidence of a rise in life change over the year and a half prior to the coronary event. Correspondingly, there was a return to baseline life change levels within a year and a half after the attack. Using a measure called Life Change Units (LCU), a sum of weighted life change events, Rahe and Paasikivi[48] found, as did others,[47,59] that quarterly LCUs averaged 20 to 30 in times of good health and rose to a level of 50 to 55 just prior to a heart attack.

In the three studies just described, subjects were asked to recall life events occurring before the cardiac event. One source of methodological concern has been that a rise in the reported number of life change events just prior to an attack may be the reflection of a more complete recall of recent events. The Rahe and Paasikivi study is reassuring on this point. Their subjects had sustained myocardial infarction during the 4 years prior to the time of data collection. However, regardless of the length of time between the attack and data collection, the rise in LCUs was in the year-quarters just prior to the infarction.

Two of the previous three studies provide evidence that the buildup of life events is not simply a normal developmental occurrence of aging that happens to coincide with, but is not causally related to, the coronary event. The Theorell and Rahe study[59] demonstrated that the life events buildup occurred only in the infarction group and not in the group of healthy control persons. The Rahe and Paasikivi study[48] showed that the buildup tapered off and returned to the low baseline of LCUs before the attack, suggesting that the buildup was illness related and not simply an artifact of normal aging.

In 1973 and 1974, Rahe et al. published reports of work on much larger groups of Finnish survivors of myocardial infarction (n = 279) and victims of sudden death (n = 226).[50,51] In this culturally distinct population, findings strikingly similar to those already described in the Swedish groups were obtained. LCUs were found to increase significantly in the 6 months before both sudden cardiac death and nonfatal myocardial infarction. These results held for subjects with and without illness experience prior to the coronary event. The latter finding counters the alternative explanation that LCUs may increase because of premonitory cardiac symptoms. But these results do confirm that individuals experiencing additional health problems have elevated LCU scores. This research project also developed data that showed that women victims of coronary disease experienced a life change buildup similar to that of men. Further, comparisons of survivors and their spouses indicated that moderately good agreement existed regarding report of recent life events, an important finding given our dependence on reports of spouses for life change information about nonsurvivors.

A 1975 study by Lundberg et al.[36] of 56 Swedish survivors of myocardial infarction and 33 matched control subjects replicated the findings of earlier retrospective studies that life changes rise before the attack. Using a variety of methods for calculating life events scores, they found that the best prediction of infarction was obtained when each individual rated for himself the degree of "upsettingness" of each life change event experienced as compared with the usual external consensus estimates of the degree of adjustment required by each event. However, even the latter approach to scoring resulted in the expected rise of events scores prior to illness.

In an attempt to gain greater control of possible genetic and environmental factors in this type of study, Ulf[62] studied nine pairs of monozygotic and eighteen pairs of dizygotic twins, one partner of which had died of coronary disease. Using the familiar retrospective approach, deceased twins had experienced higher life change levels over the 4 years prior to the coronary death, though only monozygotic nonsurvivors were significantly higher than their surviving twins. At variance with previous studies was the finding that both survivor and nonsurvivor of the nine monozygotic pairs showed a tendency to have a buildup of life changes prior to the time of the fatal event. No explanation was offered, albeit small sample size lowers confidence in the stability of this result. Ulf examined life events to see if any particular type of change stood out as a predictor of the coronary event; as in other studies,[35,52,57] it was found that a work-related event was significantly discriminative of a cardiac event.

A 1975 study by Theorell and Rahe[60] compared eighteen coronary death victims with eighteen survivors of myocardial infarction. Using only medical chart entries by physicians as a source of information on life events, a peak of life change events was found in the coronary death group at 1 year before death. Contrary to earlier results, no peak was found for survivors of an infarction. These chart reviews provided life events data recorded by a "neutral" observer prior to the death of the patient. It is encouraging that even these incomplete data tend to support earlier results for one group of subjects. Theorell and Rahe point out that the peaking phenomenon may be caused, in part, by the buildup of health problems in the last year of life. While this explanation no doubt applies, results of other studies[7,47,50,59] show the buildup of life events even when health status was controlled.

In 1976, Theorell[58] reported on a 2-year study in which 200 healthy construction workers were questioned about life change and chronic life "discord" experienced in the previous year and then were followed for 2 years to ascertain health change information. While only two instances of myocardial infarction occurred in the group, hypertension was a cardiovascular endpoint sufficient in prevalence for study. The group classified as high discord (indicating chronic life dissatisfaction and disruption) and high life change demonstrated significantly more hypertension than any other group. Neither life change nor discord alone was associated with elevated blood pressure. Since the number of infarctions was small, it is not possible to compare this study with the others reviewed above, especially in terms of mounting life changes.

In 1976, Rahe et al.[52] conducted a comparison study of East and West Finns. Their interest in comparing these two groups stemmed from the substantially higher coronary disease rates in East Finland. In light of the depressed economy in the East, the disruption caused by Soviet annexation of nearby, formerly Finnish land, and substantial emigration of its youth, life events scores were expected to be higher than in the West. This expectation was fulfilled although survivors of infarctions, whether East or West in origin, showed similar levels of life change elevations before coronary attack. As was detected in studies described above, LCUs rose two to three times over comparable baseline levels the previous year. Likewise, survivors had life change levels about twice that of their healthy counterparts. While no direct link can be drawn from these data between the high levels of life change of East Finns and their higher incidence of heart disease, the data certainly suggest that this possibility should be considered.

Finally, in a very cautiously conducted 1976 study, Connolly[7] found higher life change scores in survivors of infarction than in matched healthy control subjects in the final 3 weeks before the attack. When only subjects with a sudden onset of infarction, without anginal prodromata, were considered, differences between patients and control subjects were found not only in the last 3 weeks but also in the entire 12 weeks prior to the attack. Although the study design called for retrospective assessment of life events, Connolly was careful to include only events that were unlikely to be a result of illness itself. He was also careful to separate subjects with long-term symptoms of angina from those with a sudden, unheralded onset of illness. Similarly, no assumptions about the additivity of life events were made, but instead the subject was coded simply as life events present or absent. Given this highly prudent approach to data collection and analysis, it is impressive that earlier results are largely supported.

Findings regarding the association between life events on the one hand and coronary disease and sudden death on the other may now be summarized:

1. There is support for the proposition that life change events increase prior to cardiac illness, although the lead-time between events peaks and illness varies with reports between 2 years and 3 weeks.
2. Retrospective study designs dominate the literature and leave open the possibility of biased recall on the part of the cardiac subjects and their spouses. This may falaciously appear to confirm the life events–health change hypothesis. However, several researchers have taken steps to neutralize this threat and still have found support for the hypothesis.

It should be evident from the foregoing review that most research efforts have thus far been expended trying to prove the existence of an association between life change and cardiac illness. Factors that mediate such a relationship have not been examined, nor have factors that might predispose to increasing life change been sufficiently explored. While it is appropriate that such research should follow the establishment of clear links between life events and illness outcome, the time seems to have arrived for work on these aspects of the process. Finally, studies of physical factors that may mediate the life events–health change relationship are needed and, in fact, have already begun. This is the topic of the following section.

POSSIBLE LINKING MECHANISMS

Life events and coronary risk factors

The literature pertinent to recent life events is particularly meager regarding their relationship to coronary risk factors for two reasons: (1) until recently life events were not considered pathogenic for heart disease and (2) life events tend to be viewed as an acute precipitating factor in myocardial infarction and sudden death rather than as a chronic predisposing factor in coronary disease per se.* Regarding the second point, most risk factors for atherosclerotic heart disease such as smoking, hypertension, and elevated serum cholesterol levels are viewed as operating over extended periods to promote vascular damage and plaque production in the coronary arteries. Life events, on the other hand, are seen as being more nearly like acute physical exertion in the way it causes excessive demand for cardiac work (output). Though life events seem to accrue over several months prior to the attack, most discussions in the literature view this factor as a cause of increasing psychophysiological strain that generates more demand for cardiac work than the coronary and conductive systems can support. Hence it has not

*See Rahe and Lind,[47] Rahe et al.[50] Theorell,[56,57] and Theorell and Rahe.[59]

seemed appropriate to many investigators to examine the relationships between life events and the classic coronary risk factors.

In 1972, Theorell et al.[61] reported a study of week-to-week variations in LCUs and several serum metabolites believed to be associated with both behavioral responses and coronary disease. They included cholesterol, triglycerides, and uric acid levels. None of these metabolites were significantly related to LCUs, although (as will be described below) life change was correlated significantly with catecholamine levels.

In 1976, two further studies appeared that were able to look at the relationships between life change and selected risk factors for coronary disease. Rahe et al.[52] in their study comparing East and West Finns, explored the association between risk factors and incidence of coronary disease, as well as the prevalence of these risk factors in the two populations. As expected, both systolic and diastolic blood pressures were correlated with incidence. Cholesterol was significantly related only among East Finns. Neither smoking nor body mass was predictive of coronary disease in either group of Finns. The East Finns, known to sustain a higher incidence of coronary disease, smoked more and had higher cholesterol levels and higher systolic blood pressures than did West Finns. Life change intensity failed to correlate significantly with any risk factor except for a marginal association with systolic pressure in East Finns. These data, along with those discussed in the previous section describing the buildup of life change in these individuals, seem to suggest that classic risk factors and life change are independent of one another in their impact on coronary outcome.

A risk factor study by Theorell[57] also indicated that life change is not related to the coronary risk factors described above (smoking behavior was not reported). However, it was learned that subjects with high life change who have high chronic "discord" scores displayed significantly higher blood pressure than other subject categories. This relationship was strongest in younger subjects, 41 to 46 years of age. In general these three studies[52,57,61] give little indication that life events either influence or are influenced by the traditional cardiac risk factors.

Life events and type A behavior

In the context of risk factors, evidence was presented in the previous chapter that a behavioral complex referred to as type A behavior pattern might be considered as predictive of coronary artery disease. What is the relationship between life events buildup and type A behavior? While this question has not been the subject of empirical research to date, several authors[57,62] have considered this question at a theoretical level. As mentioned previously, there is consensus that life events act to precipitate or trigger coronary events, although this may range from a few days to a few years. Type A behavior, on the other hand, is generally viewed as acting over many years and contributing to the progression of the underlying atherosclerotic disease process in a way analogous to that of chronically elevated cholesterol and/or blood pressure.

If both life events and type A behavior ultimately prove to be influential in production of coronary disease, it will be of interest to define their interrelationship. Are these factors totally independent of one another in the impact on this disease? It is also possible that type A individuals in their drive to accumulate, compete, and produce at high levels of intensity tend to expose themselves to more life change than would be true of type B individuals. For example, the type A person may change jobs, residences, and many correlated life patterns in an effort to support his achievement drive. In this sense, type A behavior is itself a determinant of life change. Reversing the causal direction, it is conceivable that high levels of life change trigger type A behavior as a coping mechanism. The person thrown into a position of great work responsibility may find that the type A pattern of increased rapidity of action and deliberate control of distraction are quite helpful, instrumental responses in the short run. Only future research will clarify the links, if any, between these two behavioral factors.

Life events, catecholamines, and cardiac function

Research into the psychophysiological mechanisms that promote translation of recent life experience into cardiac events is still needed. An example presented earlier in this chapter, regarding the negative cardiovascular effects of transfers from coronary care unit to convalescent ward, hinted at one possible research direction, namely the role of catecholamine excretion as mediator. In that study, the strain of transfer was manifested in elevated excretion levels; presumably, these in turn produced cardiac complications. That study is one of a group of studies that shows the stress responsiveness of epinephrine (adrenaline) and norepinephrine (noradrenaline) levels in cardiac patients[29,63] and well individuals.[13] Theorell et al.[61] have cited "experiments on humans (that) have demonstrated that the catecholamine output increases in situations that are *novel* to the subject."[15,34] It has also been suggested that, whether coping with desirable or undesirable life changes, systematic variations in catecholamines are likely.[16,34]

In a study of 21 male survivors of infarction, Theorell[57,61] found that catecholamine levels were significantly elevated in subjects with elevations in life change. The relationship between life change and epinephrine was stronger than that between life change and norepinephrine. The latter finding is in agreement with those of Frankenhauser and Johannsson[13,14] that epinephrine excretion is more sensitive to psychological stress than is norepinephrine.

One final study that appears to speak to the issue of mechanisms linking life events and coronary disease is that of Theorell and Rahe.[60] In a study of 36 male and female victims of myocardial infarction, eighteen surviving and eighteen not, it was found that the nonsurviving group experienced buildups of both LCUs 1 year before their attack and ventricular contractile force at about 6 months before the attack. The surviving individuals experienced neither. Although the meaning of these findings is not totally clear, one interpretation is that life changes stimulate psychophysiological strain that results in signs of impending cardiac failure.

SUMMARY

This chapter presented evidence that significant life events may precipitate cardiac illness and sudden death. In the first section, accounts were presented of sudden cardiac death that seemed to occur soon after single traumatic events. These events usually involved instances of loss and fear, although accounts of death after triumph and exaltation were also found. Several psychophysiological theories were suggested that may begin to explain the mechanisms leading to such deaths. These included the sympathetic mechanism in which extreme arousal may result in cardiac acceleration and rhythm disturbances and the mechanism of parasympathetic dominance in which cardiac deceleration likewise results in arrhythmias.

The origins of the life events–health change theory were traced to the works of Cannon and Selye, both early researchers in the field of psychosomatic medicine. By the 1950s, Holmes had developed the life events–health change paradigm into a specific area of research and theory within the psychosomatic field. In the past 30 years, the validity of the model has found support in its application to subjects of several nationalities experiencing a variety of physical and emotional health problems, both minor and severe. The quality of research has also been improving with a shift from the methodologically weaker retrospective study designs to stronger prospective ones. Although numerous problems remain, as critics in the area attest, guarded optimism persists that the paradigm will be borne out and strengthened with further research. Major efforts are still needed in gaining an understanding of the factors that promote and inhibit the translation of life change experience into illness.

Literature was reviewed that appears to link the accumulation of various life changes with coronary disease, especially myocardial infarction and sudden death. Substantial agreement was found that life events accumulate and peak at some point prior to cardiac symptomatology. The peak has been reported to occur between 2 years and a few weeks before the cardiac event. There is agreement that the life change buildup should be viewed as a precipitating force rather than a chronic predisposing one. Sources of possible bias in these data were discussed, such as selective recall of life changes and the effects of premonitory symptoms of cardiovascular illness. Evidence in the research literature regarding the mechanisms that may link behavior and disease were shown to be sparse, but some data suggesting the mediating role of catecholamine excretions were presented.

REFERENCES

1. Alexander, F.: Psychosomatic medicine: its principles and applications, New York, 1950, W. W. Norton Co.
2. Alverez, W.: Dying of fright, Mod. Med. **35:**69, 1967.
3. Bramwell, S.: Personality and psychosocial variables in college athletics, Medical thesis, Seattle, 1971, University of Washington.
4. Cannon, W.: Bodily changes in pain, hunger, fear and rage, New York, 1929, Appleton-Century-Crofts.
5. Cannon, W.: The wisdom of the body, New York, 1939, W. W. Norton Co.
6. Cannon, W.: Voodoo death, Am. Anthropol. **44:**169, 1942.
7. Connolly, J.: Life events before myocardial infarction, J. Hum. Stress **2:**3, 1976.
8. Earls, J., and Wolf, S.: A report of multiple periodic anniversary reactions in one individual, Ann. Intern. Med. **58:**530, 1963.
9. Eckenhoff, J.: Some preoperative warnings of potential operating room deaths, N. Engl. J. Med. **255:**1075, 1956.
10. Engel, G.: Sudden and rapid death during psychological stress, Ann. Intern. Med. **74:** 771, 1971.
11. Fischer, H., and Dlin, B.: Man's determination of his time of illness or death: anniversary reactions and emotional deadlines, Geriatrics **25:**83, 1971.
12. Fitzhugh, G., and Hamilton, B.: Coronary occlusion and fatal angina pectoris, J.A.M.A. **100:**475, 1933.
13. Frankenhauser, M.: Behavior and circulating catecholamines, Brain Res. **31:**142, 1971.
14. Frankenhauser, M., and Johannson, G.: Task demand as reflected in catecholamine excretion and heart rate, J. Hum. Stress **2:**15, 1976.
15. Frankenhauser, M., et al.: Catecholamine excretion as related to cognitive and emotional reaction patterns, Psychosom. Med. **30:**109, 1968.
16. Fröberg, J., et al.: Physiological and biochemical stress reactions induced by psychosocial stimuli. In Levi, L., editor: Society, stress, and disease, New York, 1971, Oxford University Press.
17. Garrity, T., Somes, G., and Marx, M.: The relationship of personality life change, psychophysiological strain and health status in a college population, Soc. Sci. Med. **11:**257, 1977.
18. Gazes, P., Sovell, B., and Dellastatious, J.: Continuous radioelectric-cardiographic monitoring of football coaches during games, Am. Heart J. **78:**509, 1969.
19. Gellhorn, E.: Principles of autonomic-somatic integrations, Minneapolis, 1967, University of Minnesota Press.
20. Hamburg, D.: Plasma and urinary corticoid levels in naturally occurring psychological stresses, Res. Publ. Assoc. Res. Nerv. Ment. Dis. Proc. **40:**406, 1962.
21. Hanson, J., and Tabakin, B.: Electrocardiographic telemetry in skiers. Anticipatory and recovery heart rate during competition, N. Engl. J. Med. **271:**181, 1964.
22. Harmon, D., Masuda, M., and Holmes, T.: The social readjustment scale: a cross-cultural study of Western Europeans and Americans, J. Psychosom. Res. **14:**391, 1970.
23. Helpern, M., and Rabson, S.: Sudden and unexpected natural death, Am. J. Med. Sci. **220:**262, 1950.
24. Holmes, T., and Masuda, M.: Life change and illness susceptibility. In Dohrenwend, B. S., and Dohrenwend, B. P., editors: Stressful life events, New York, 1974, John Wiley & Sons, Inc.
25. Holmes, T., and Rahe, R.: The social readjustment rating scale, J. Psychosom. Res. **11:**213, 1967.
26. Holmes, T., et al.: The nose. An experimental study of reactions within the nose in human subjects during varying life experiences, Springfield, Ill., 1950, Charles C Thomas, Publisher.
27. James, T.: QT prolongation and sudden death, Mod. Concepts Cardiovasc. Dis. **38:** 35, 1969.
28. James, T., Froggatt, P., and Marshall, T.: Sudden death in young athletes, Ann. Intern. Med. **67:**1013, 1967.
29. Januszewicz, W., et al.: Urinary excretion of free norepinephrine and free epinephrine in patients with acute myocardial infarction in relation to its clinical course, Am. Heart J. **76:**345, 1968.
30. Jarvinen, K.: Can ward rounds be a danger to patients with myocardial infarction? Br. Med. J. **1:**318, 1955.

31. Klein, R., et al.: Transfer from a coronary care unit, Arch. Intern. Med. **122:**104, 1968.
32. Klein, R., et al.: Urinary catecholamine excretion in patients with myocardial infarction, Arch. Intern. Med. **122:**476, 1968.
33. Kuller, L., Lilienfeld, A., and Fisher, R.: Epidemiological study of sudden and unexpected deaths in adults, Medicine **46:**341, 1967.
34. Levi, L.: The urinary output of the adrenaline and noradrenaline during pleasant and unpleasant emotional states, Psychosom. Med. **27:**80, 1965.
35. Liljefors, I., and Rahe, R.: An identical twin study of psychosocial factors in coronary heart disease, Psychosom. Med. **32:**523, 1970.
36. Lundberg, U., Theorell, T., and Lind, E.: Life changes and myocardial infarction: individual differences in life change scaling, J. Psychosom. Res. **19:**27, 1975.
37. Mason, J.: A review of psychoendocrine research on sympathetic-adrenal medullary system, Psychosom. Med. **30:**631, 1968.
38. Mason, J., et al.: Concurrent measurement of 17-hydroxycorticosteroids and pepsinogen levels during prolonged emotional stress in the monkey, Psychosom. Med. **21:**432, 1959.
39. Masuda, M., and Holmes, T.: The social readjustment rating scale: a cross-cultural study of Japanese and Americans, J. Psychosom. Res. **11:**227, 1967.
40. McConnell, J.: Discussion of Yawger, N.: Emotions as the cause of rapid and sudden death, Arch. Neurol. Psychiatry **36:**879, 1936.
41. Moss, A., and Wynar, B.: Tachycardia in house officers presenting cases at grand rounds, Ann. Intern. Med. **72:**255, 1970.
42. Moss, G.: Illness, immunity and social interaction, New York, 1973, John Wiley & Sons, Inc.
43. Rabb, W.: Cardiotoxic biochemical effects of emotional-environmental stresses—fundamentals of psychocardiology. In Levi, L., editor: Society, stress, and disease, New York, 1971, Oxford University Press.
44. Rabkin, J., and Streuning, E.: Life events, stress and illness, Science **194:**1013, 1974.
45. Rahe, R.: Life change measurement as a predictor of illness, Proc. R. Soc. Med. **61:**1124, 1968.
46. Rahe, R.: The pathway between subject's recent life changes and their near-future illness reports: representative results and methodological issues. In Dohrenwend, B. S., and Dohrenwend, B. P., editors: Stressful life events, New York, 1974, John Wiley & Sons, Inc.
47. Rahe, R., and Lind, E.: Psychosocial factors and sudden cardiac death: a pilot study, J. Psychosom. Res. **15:**19, 1971.
48. Rahe, R., and Paasikivi, J.: Psychosocial factors and myocardial infarction. II. An outpatient study in Sweden, J. Psychosom. Res. **15:**33, 1971.
49. Rahe, R., et al.: Subjects' life changes, symptom recognition and illness reports in the Norwegian Navy. Unit Report, San Diego, 1973, U.S. Navy Medical Neuropsychiatric Research Unit.
50. Rahe, R., et al.: Subjects' recent life changes and coronary heart disease in Finland, Am. J. Psychiatry **130:**1222, 1973.
51. Rahe, R., et al.: Recent life changes, myocardial infarction, and abrupt coronary death, Arch. Intern. Med. **133:**221, 1974.
52. Rahe, R., et al.: Recent life changes and coronary heart disease in East versus West Finland, J. Psychosom. Res. **20:**431, 1976.
53. Selye, H.: The stress of life, New York, 1965, McGraw-Hill Book Co.
54. Spain, D., Bradess, V., and Mohr, C.: Coronary atherosclerosis as a cause of unexpected and unexplained death. An autopsy study from 1949-1959, J.A.M.A. **174:**384, 1960.
55. Sudnow, D.: Passing on, Englewood Cliffs, N.J., 1967, Prentice-Hall, Inc.
56. Theorell, T.: Psychosocial factors in relation to the onset of myocardial infarction and to some metabolic variables—a pilot study. Academic thesis, Karolinska Institute, 1970.
57. Theorell, T.: Life events before and after the onset of a premature myocardial infarction. In Dohrenwend, B. S., and Dohrenwend, B. P., editors: Stressful life events, New York, 1974, John Wiley & Sons, Inc.
58. Theorell, T.: Selected illnesses and somatic factors in relation to two psychosocial stress indices—a prospective study on middle-aged construction building workers, J. Psychosom. Res. **20:**7, 1976.
59. Theorell, T., and Rahe, R.: Psychosocial factors and myocardial infarction. I. An inpatient study in Sweden, J. Psychosom. Res. **15:**25, 1971.

60. Theorell, T., and Rahe, R.: Life change events, ballistocardiography and coronary death, J. Hum. Stress **1:**18, 1975.
61. Theorell, T., et al.: A longitudinal study of 21 subjects with coronary heart disease: life changes, catecholamine excretion and related biochemical reactions, Psychosom. Med. **34:**505, 1972.
62. Ulf, D.: Life change patterns prior to death in ischemic heart disease. A study on death-discordant twins, J. Psychosom. Res. **19:**273, 1975.
63. Valori, C., Thomas, M., and Shillingford, J.: Free noradrenaline and adrenaline excretion in relation to clinical syndromes following myocardial infarction, Am. J. Cardiol. **20:**605, 1967.
64. Warner, W.: A black civilization, New York, 1937, Harper & Row, Publishers.
65. Wolff, H.: Protective reaction patterns and disease, Ann. Intern. Med. **27:**944, 1947.
66. Woon, R., et al.: The social readjustment rating scale: a cross-cultural study of Malaysians and Americans, J. Cross-Cultural Psychol. **2:**373, 1971.
67. Yawger, N.: Emotions as the cause of rapid and sudden death, Arch. Neurol. Psychiatry **36:**875, 1936.

3

Physiological mechanisms underlying the association between psychosocial factors and coronary disease

REDFORD B. WILLIAMS, Jr.

The first two chapters have dealt with the association between certain psychological and social factors and an increased risk of suffering the clinical manifestations of coronary disease. Unfortunately, the mere fact of association between certain risk factors and the disease does not permit the inference of a causal relationship. To assume causality, it must be possible also to show increased risk with the addition of the risk factor in question and decreased risk with removal of the factor. The necessity of identifying true causal relationships is not a trivial issue, for only when this has been accomplished is it possible to discover rational prevention and treatment measures. As stated in Chapter 1, the type A behavior pattern is associated with increased subsequent risk of suffering such clinical coronary events as myocardial infarction and sudden death. A key question suggested by this association concerns the underlying mechanism. Does type A behavior result in increased coronary events by precipitating thrombosis or other catastrophic events in individuals already at risk as a result of preexisting coronary atherosclerosis? Or does type A behavior contribute to coronary atherosclerosis itself in a more direct fashion? There is now emerging evidence that type A individuals exhibit more extreme coronary atherosclerosis as documented by coronary arteriography.[78] This evidence has important implications not only for understanding causal mechanisms but also for intervention strategies. It suggests that attempts to reduce the impact of psychosocial factors on coronary disease risk should be an integral part of early primary prevention efforts as well as programs of secondary prevention and rehabilitation. Lest the reader assume that the case for a causal role of psychosocial factors in coronary disease is weaker

Supported in part by Research Scientist Development Award K01-MH-70482, National Institute of Mental Health.

than the case for the various physical risk factors (blood pressure, serum cholesterol levels, and cigarette smoking), it is worth recalling that at the present time there has been no association conclusively proved between a decrease in any of the physical risk factors and a decline in the risk of coronary disease. For example, results of the Veterans Administration Collaborative Study[15] indicate that lowering elevated blood pressure is associated with a decrease in the incidence of strokes but *not* of myocardial infarction. Thus we still are unsure of the mechanisms underlying the association between risk factors and coronary disease.

In this chapter, I shall attempt to identify mechanisms that may explain the association between psychosocial factors and the risk of coronary disease. Most of the previous work in this area has been directed toward demonstrating the existence of the association between the two. The question now arises regarding the basis of this association. As we seek to answer this question, the reader is warned that what follows, although based on sound research, must be viewed as speculation, just as the supposition that high blood pressure causes coronary disease via a mechanism of injuring arterial walls or altering smooth muscle metabolism is also speculation. This chapter is provided in an effort to increase understanding of the nature of the association between psychosocial risk factors and coronary disease and to provide an overview of the type of work that will be required in the future to exploit clinically what we know concerning that association.

Insofar as psychosocial factors cause coronary disease, it is likely that this occurs via effects on the physiology of the cardiovascular system, on lipid metabolism, or on some combination of the two. That is, the link between a certain behavior pattern and the occurrence of a pathological lesion in the coronary vasculature must involve effects of the behavior in question on intervening factors responsible for the initiation and development of the atheromatous plaque. Current thinking holds that the initiating lesion in coronary disease, the atheromatous plaque, develops as a result of mechanical injury to the endothelial lining and/or smooth muscle wall of the artery involved.[25] Increased levels of circulating lipids also play a role.[26] What follows, therefore, is a review of means by which psychosocial factors might contribute to vascular injury and to altered lipid metabolism. First, we shall consider studies in animals and humans that demonstrate a relationship between various behaviors and changes in cardiovascular function and lipid metabolism that could lead to vascular injury and thus to an increased incidence of coronary disease. Second, to indicate that such relationships have an anatomical and neurophysiological basis, we shall consider studies of central nervous system control of cardiovascular function and lipid metabolism. Third, to indicate the peripheral neurophysiological bases of behavioral and social influences, studies of the sympathetic nervous system as a mediator of stress effects will be reviewed. Fourth, since psychosocial factors are prevalent in a much larger population than eventually develops coronary disease, we shall consider studies of individual differences in perceptual style that might modify the effect of psychosocial factors on cardiovascular function and lipid metabolism. Finally, a concluding section will present speculations concerning how the foregoing might be applied in planning rational preventive and treatment approaches.

PHYSIOLOGICAL CORRELATES OF BEHAVIOR

A number of studies using animal models have shown that both acute and long-term changes in cardiovascular function occur in association with various behavioral manipulations. Benson et al.[6] found that monkeys required to press a key to avoid painful shocks developed blood pressure elevations to average levels of 168 mm Hg. The blood pressure remained significantly elevated even after the termination of the experiment. Anderson et al.[4,5] observed increases in blood pressure and total peripheral resistance and decreases in heart rate and cardiac output in dogs during the hour prior to an avoidance experiment similar to that conducted by Benson et al.[6] In a study of the cardiovascular responses of monkeys to avoidance behavior carried out over periods of 2 to 14 months, Forsyth and Harris[13] were able to produce blood pressure elevations that were sustained throughout the day and not just during the avoidance behavior. The increased blood pressure was associated with a decrease in total peripheral resistance and an increase in cardiac output, with the cardiac output increase being shunted away from skin, gastrointestinal tract, and kidneys to the skeletal muscles and heart. In contrast to the elevated cardiac output and decreased peripheral resistance with shunting of blood to the skeletal musculature that Forsyth and Harris[13] observed during the stress of shock avoidance, Adams et al.[3] observed a decreased cardiac output and shunting of blood away from the skeletal musculature in cats during preparation for fighting.

The need for caution in identifying the specific nature of the behavior leading to a specific pattern of cardiovascular response that is suggested by the animal studies becomes even more apparent when one considers studies linking behavior and cardiovascular function in man. There is an extensive literature concerning the relationship between stress and cardiovascular function in man. Using mental arithmetic (with or without accompanying harrassment by the experimenter) as the stressor, a number of investigators have observed a rather consistent pattern of cardiovascular response consisting of increased cardiac output, decreased total peripheral resistance, and shunting of blood away from the skin and viscera to the skeletal musculature, as shown in Fig. 3.[2,9,44] This pattern is similar to that observed by Forsyth and Harris[13] in monkeys during avoidance behavior. As in the animal experiments, however, the picture is not as simple in man as this description would suggest. For example, Lacey et al.[28] have shown that in addition to the heart rate increases observed when individuals want to shut

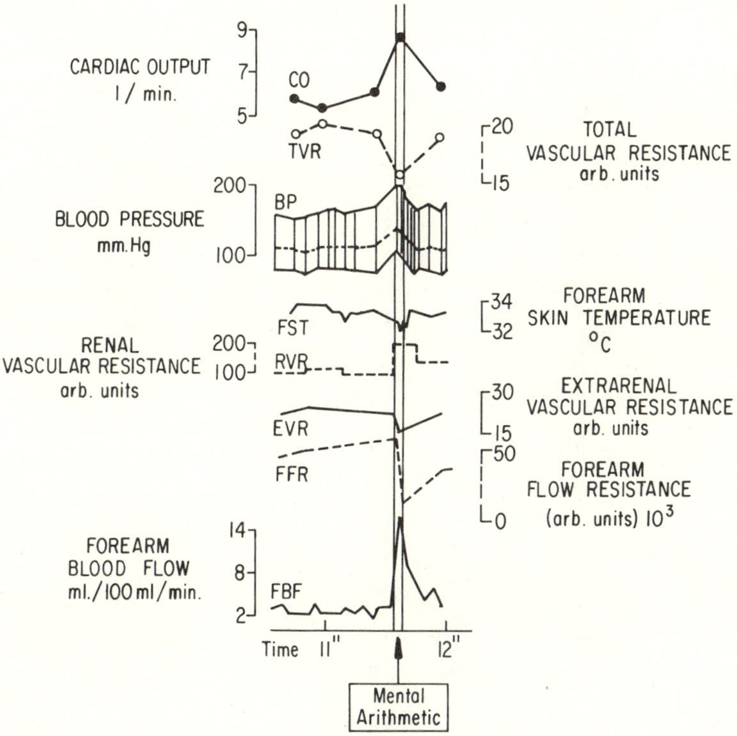

Fig. 3. Hemodynamic responses in various vascular beds to stress of doing mental arithmetic. (From Brod, J., et al.: Clin. Sci. **18:**269, 1959.)

out distracting environmental stimuli (as, for example, when solving a mental arithmetic problem), the heart rate slows when an individual is trying to note and detect environmental stimuli. While noting the phenomenon of a decreased heart rate during sensory intake, Obrist et al.[35] also note a decrease in ongoing skeletal muscle activity. The heart rate slows whenever an individual intends to take in sensory information, even when it may be as unpleasant as pictures of homicide victims.[10]

The discovery of a behavioral-cardiovascular relationship different from the classical pattern of stress in association with increased cardiac output and shunting of blood to muscle might not be so important in relation to coronary disease, were it not for more recent evidence that sensory intake behavior has more complex cardiovascular effects than simple heart rate slowing. In addition, sensory intake behavior is also associated with vasoconstriction in skeletal muscle.[7,52] As shown in Fig. 4, sensory intake behavior is associated with an increase in forearm vascular resistance, while sensory rejection behavior is associated with

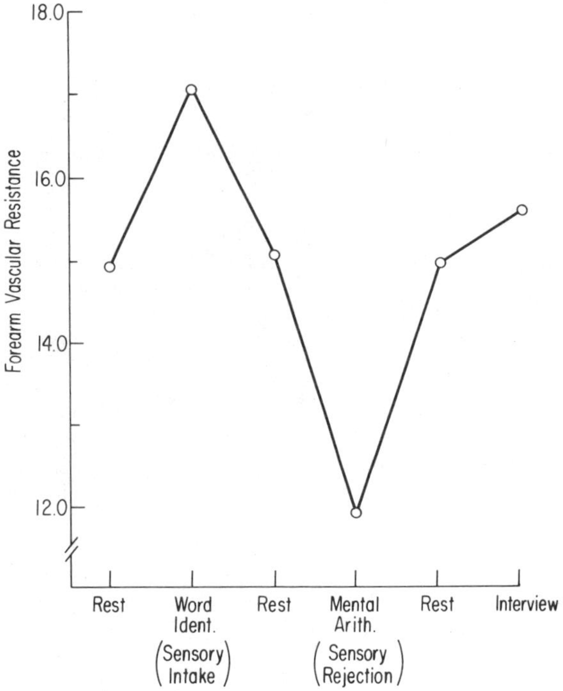

Fig. 4. Changes in forearm vascular resistance measured during sensory intake behavior and sensory rejection behavior.

a vasodilation. The vasoconstriction occurs whether the sensory intake behavior is required of the individual by the demands of the situation or is chosen by him in a situation permitting free choice of sensory intake or sensory rejection behavior. There is a significant increase in levels of plasma catecholamines in association with sensory intake behavior,[51] a phenomenon that will later be shown to be important in the risk of coronary disease.

Friedman et al.[16] have shown that lipid metabolism levels also respond to life stresses. Accountants manifested significant serum cholesterol increases at income tax time, the time of their most active involvement in job-related stress.

Thus it appears that a variety of behaviors are specifically associated with a variety of patterns of cardiovascular response that may be relevant to arterial injury and hence to an increased risk of coronary disease. Before proceeding to a consideration of the studies in which relationships are drawn between such response patterns and cardiovascular disease, however, a brief word is needed concerning the role and meaning of the term "stress." The work cited earlier led to the conclusion that stress is associated with an increased cardiac output and increased skeletal muscle blood flow. When behaviors other than rejection of environmental stimuli have been studied, however, it has been found that an active skeletal muscle vasoconstriction can also occur as a response to stress. The question arises, "What is stress?" Although an exhaustive consideration of this topic is beyond the scope of this chapter, certain cautionary notes are warranted. Lazarus[30] defines the occurrence of a stress reaction as dependent on the coping behavior utilized by the individual as a result of an appraisal of the potentially stressful stimulus situation. He further suggests that patterns of autonomic response must be studied to obtain a complete picture of the stress reaction, since it appears to be the *pattern* of autonomic response that reflects a "specific kind of transaction between the individual and the situation."[30] Weiner[46] indicated the importance of identifying the ". . . critical psychological stimulus with which specific physiological responses may be correlated" if we are to understand why and how different life situations give rise to different behavioral patterns that are associated in turn with different patterns of physiological response. Finally, Mason[32] suggests that it is the *behavioral response itself* that is the important intervening variable determining the physiological response to stress.

A number of studies have attempted to define the role of behavioral–cardiovascular response relationships in cardiovascular disease. Singer[43] and Harris and Singer[23] observed that young people who interacted with others in a "pressured" manner were more likely to manifest elevated blood pressure during an interview and over a follow-up period as long as 11 years. Moreover, a 5-year follow-up study demonstrated that those hypertensive patients who had interacted in a more pressured fashion suffered a higher mortality rate than those patients who interacted in a 'defended' fashion. Brod et al.[9] found that hypertensive individuals react to the stress of mental arithmetic with a more prolonged hemodynamic response and with greater renal vasoconstriction and possibly less muscle vasodilation than subjects who are normotensive. McKegney and Williams[34] found a more intense and prolonged diastolic pressor response to an interview among hypertensive than normotensive individuals. Wolf[53] has reported that patients with coronary disease show increased lability of blood pressure and that patients who die suddenly have even greater blood pressure lability than those who survive a myocardial infarction. The hemodynamic effects of such blood pressure lability could be related to arterial injury. Further implicating cardiovascular responses to everyday stimuli in the pathogenesis of coronary disease, Keys[27a] has noted that the extent of the diastolic blood pressure increase during the cold pressor test is one of the best predictors of a subsequent risk of coronary disease.

It therefore appears that in the normal day-to-day activities of attending to environmental stimuli, of shutting out stimuli to perform some mental task, and of coping or failing to cope with life stresses, individuals subject their cardiovascular systems to varying response patterns that are potentially injurious. Whether such relationships between behavior and cardiovascular response are important in the pathogenesis and course of cardiovascular disease will require extensive further research. Support for a role of such relationships in mediating the association between coronary disease and the psychological and social factors outlined in Chapters 1 and 2 is provided by a consideration of the manner in which the central and sympathetic nervous systems control the link between behavior and cardiovascular function and how individual differences in behaving and responding might be important.

CENTRAL NERVOUS SYSTEM MECHANISMS REGULATING CARDIOVASCULAR FUNCTION

Although much remains to be understood, certain brain mechanisms have been identified as mediators of behavioral-cardiovascular relationships. It is now clear that the increased cardiac output and active skeletal muscle vasodilation that occur during fight-or-flight activity (and, one might surmise, during sensory rejection behavior) are brought about by increased activity in a certain area of the hypothalamus known as the "defense area," which corresponds in many respects to the reticular activating system.[1] Animals receiving electrical stimulation in this brain area exhibit both fight-or-flight behavior and the cardiovascular pattern of increased cardiac output and skeletal muscle vasodilation. Relating possible chronic activation of this hypothalamic defense area by stress to cardiovascular disease, Folkow and Rubinstein[12] electrically stimulated the defense area in rats during a period of 4 months and observed a gradual rise in the resting blood pressure of the animals, results that suggest a possible role of such chronic effects of stress-activated defense reactions in the pathogenesis of hypertension. Williams et al. have described a blood pressure response to shock-induced fighting in rats that is mediated by peripheral sympathetic vasoconstrictor nerves.[47,48] This cardiovascular response to shock-induced fighting appears to be mediated in the brain by neurons using catecholamines as a neurotransmitter[49] and originating in a small collection of cells in the brain stem known as the locus ceruleus.[50]

Turning from brain control of cardiovascular function to control of lipid metabolism, we note that Gunn et al.[19] have found that chronic stimulation of the ventromedial nucleus of the hypothalamus of the rabbit accelerated the process of atherosclerosis induced in the animals by a diet high in cholesterol. Similarly, Gutstein et al.[20] found increased plasma triglycerides in the rat in association with stimulation of the ventromedial nucleus of the hypothalamus. Thus scientific investigation has demonstrated the existence of brain mechanisms that can mediate the effects of certain behaviors and life stress on cardiovascular function and lipid metabolism.

SYMPATHETIC NERVOUS SYSTEM EFFECTS

A number of studies have correlated the effects of psychosocial stress on sympathetic nervous system function with effects on cardiovascular function and pathology. Henry et al.[24] have found that mice subjected to chronic confrontations with other mice to obtain food develop hypertension and increased coronary atherosclerosis, which was associated with an increase in the levels of enzymes synthesizing the neurotransmitters of the sympathetic nervous system. Lamprecht et al.[29] have found that hypertension occurring in rats after chronic immobilization stress is associated with increased serum levels of dopamine-beta-hydroxylase, the enzyme that synthesizes norepinephrine.

In human beings, depression and anxiety have been correlated with increased plasma levels of the sympathetic neurotransmitter norepinephrine.[54] Frankenhauser[14] observed increased excretion of catecholamines in the urine in association with any "attention-demanding activity." In agreement with that finding, Williams et al.[51] found an increase in blood catecholamine levels during performance of a task requiring vigilance.

This increased sympathetic nervous system activity, as reflected in the various indices of catecholamine metabolism just cited, may be important for the pathogenesis or outcome of coronary disease. Raab[36] notes that both epinephrine and norepinephrine cause an increase in the consumption of oxygen by the heart, and he points out that anginal attacks have been correlated with acute, stress-induced increases in these plasma catecholamine levels. Haft et al.[21] have shown that norepinephrine infusions can cause platelet aggregation in the myocardial blood vessels of dogs, suggesting a possible role of stress-induced increases in circulating catecholamines in coronary atherosclerosis and myocardial infarction. Friedman et al.[17] found that type A men, who are prone to develop coronary disease, exhibit a larger increment in plasma norepinephrine during a problem-solving task than do type B men, who are relatively resistant to coronary disease.

ROLE OF INDIVIDUAL DIFFERENCES

Not all individuals who are subjected to life stress or who exhibit the type A behavior pattern develop coronary disease; indeed, only a small proportion do. The same statement can be made for all the physical risk factors such as serum cholesterol levels, blood pressure, and cigarette smoking. What, then, is responsible for these large individual differences in susceptibility to coronary disease? It is likely that other as yet unknown factors account for these individual differences. The foregoing discussion suggests that behavioral influences on sympathetically mediated cardiovascular responses and on lipid metabolism could play a role in determining the risk of coronary disease. The discussion that follows will consider how these behaviorally determined physiological responses, and hence the disease-related consequences, might vary from individual to individual.

Since the processing of sensory information is one important determinant of cardiovascular function, individual differences in ways of processing sensory information could account for some of the variability in the risk of coronary disease. Highlighting this possibility is the observation by Raff et al.[37] that patients who suffer a recurrent myocardial infarction within 12 weeks of their first infarct are more vigilant, hyperalert, and "overinclusive of stimulus input" than patients not suffering an early recurrence. The association of stimulus intake behavior with increased plasma catecholamine levels[51] could provide a basis—via the effects of catecholamines to increase myocardial oxygen consumption—for the increased reinfarction rate among overscanners.

One of the most widely studied measures of individual differences in perceptual style is that of field articulation. People who are field independent (FI) are able to orient a rod to the true vertical on the rod and frame test, while field-dependent (FD) individuals are distracted by the surrounding frame and never get the rod oriented as closely to the true vertical as the field-independent individuals. FI and FD persons differ in terms of cardiovascular and metabolic responses to a number of stimuli in ways that might have relevance to the risk of coronary disease. FI subjects show a greater heart rate and blood pressure increase in response to insulin hypoglycemia than do FD subjects.[42] On the other hand, FD subjects show a greater range of lipid mobilization response to the stress of an intravenous saline injection[33] and also exhibit greater degrees of venoconstriction during rest periods.[41] The heart rate slowing during sensory intake, which was described in the first section of this chapter,[10,28,35] is exhibited to a greater degree by FI rather than FD subjects.[18]

Another measure of how an individual habitually processes sensory information is described by the augmenting and reducing phenomenon. "Augmenters" are those who increase the size of their average cortical evoked potentials to light flashes as the flashes increase in intensity. "Reducers," on the other hand, decrease the size of their evoked potentials as stimulus intensity increases. Schechter and Buchsbaum[40] have shown that augmenters are persons who habitually do not attend to their sensory environment, while reducers are habitually attending. Williams et al.[51] found that reducers (or habitual attenders) have a significantly higher resting skeletal muscle vasomotor tone than augmenters (or nonattenders). In addition, people who exhibit evoked potential patterns indicative of a high level of ability to focus their attention also have higher levels of sympathetic nervous system activity (as indexed by serum levels of dopamine-beta-hydroxylase, the enzyme converting dopamine into norepinephrine) than those whose evoked potential patterns indicated less ability to focus attention on external stimuli.[51]

In terms of individual differences in lipid metabolism as related to psychosocial factors, Thomas[45] observed in a prospective study of medical students an association between a tendency to react to stress with increased activity and exhilaration and the presence of hypercholesteremia. Type A individuals, who are prone to myocardial infarction, tend to have higher serum cholesterol levels.[16,37] Harlan et al.,[22] in the "Thousand Aviator Study," found that subjects whose scores on the Guilford-Zimmerman Temperament Survey suggested a high level of aggression also have higher levels of serum lipoproteins, triglycerides, and cholesterol than subjects without such scores.

Thus, individual differences in perceptual styles—in how individuals habitually process the stimulus inputs from their sensory environment—can be clearly related to sympathetic nervous system function. Moreover, these relationships are in agreement with the concept that different patterns of sensory processing are associated with distinctly different patterns of sympathetic nervous system response. That is, persons with a perceptual style suggestive of sensory rejection (augmenters) show skeletal muscle forearm blood flow hemodynamics similar to those associated with sensory rejection behavior, while persons with a perceptual style suggestive of sensory intake (reducers) manifest a hemodynamic pattern similar to that elicited by sensory intake behavior.

These individual differences in perceptual style could account for some of the relationships between certain psychosocial factors and the risk of coronary disease. Do type A individuals go through their day in a hypervigilant, overscanning perceptual mode? On the basis of published descriptions of type A characteristics, it might be concluded that such is indeed to be expected. If so, then the sympathetic nervous system correlates of such behavior could be expected to subject the cardiovascular system of type A individuals to greater physical loads and stresses day in and day out, thus providing the intervening links between the personality-behavior pattern and coronary disease pathogenesis. Preliminary studies by Dembyoski et al.[11] and by Manuck et al.[31] do suggest that heart rate and blood pressure responses are more marked in young type A males during challenging perceptual-motor and cognitive tasks.

PREVENTION AND TREATMENT OF CORONARY DISEASE

"In spite of all advances in diagnosis and treatment, prevention is essential for any real control over most of the heart disease problem."[27] Keys has also suggested that prevention could consist in controlling such physical risk factors as high serum cholesterol and blood pressure levels. As noted earlier, the studies conducted to date in which control of these risk factors has been achieved have not demonstrated a concomitant decline in the incidence of coronary disease. Thus far there have been no systematic, large-scale studies in which the object has been to assess the effect of controlling psychosocial risk factors on the risk of coronary disease. Not only is *prevention* of coronary disease essential if we are to achieve any "real control over most of the heart disease problem,"[27] but it is only

Table 2. Summary of possible mediating factors in the association between behavior and coronary disease

	Behavior	Associated perceptual style	Associated cardivascular response pattern	Peripheral sympathetic mediation	CNS mediation	Possible effects on heart	Possible intervention
Life ↗	Sensory intake; ? hypervigilance, overscanning	Reducer ? Field dependent ? More intense in type A	Decreased heart rate Skeletal muscle vasoconstriction	α-Adrenergic, norepinephrine released by peripheral sympathetic nerves	Increased sympathetic outflow; ? from posterior hypothalamus; requires intact CNS catecholamines	Increased work load caused by increased peripheral resistance Norepinephrine leads to increased metabolic rate in heart	Biofeedback training to decrease vasoconstriction Sympatholytic medication (e.g., α-blocking agent) Modify behavior
stresses ↘	Sensory rejection; ? anxiety, denial	Augmenter ? Field independent ?More intense in type A	Increased heart rate Skeletal muscle vasodilation	β-Adrenergic, epinephrine released by adrenal medulla	Activation of hypothalamic "defense" center in reticular activating system	Increased work load caused by increased cardiac output Possible hemodynamic injury to coronary arteries	Biofeedback training to decrease heart rate β-blocking agent (propranolol) Modify behavior

by demonstrating that control of a given risk factor decreases risk that we can identify causal mechanisms.

Although methods of psychological intervention such as the use of group therapy in the rehabilitation of coronary patients are now beginning,[38] the obstacles to demonstrating the efficacy of these approaches are considerable. Until the intervening mechanisms are identified with some accuracy, investigators are in the position of "removing the pump handle" to halt the cholera epidemic, instead of taking more cost-effective measures to deal with the causative bacteria. How might knowledge of the factors identified as potential mediators of the association between psychosocial factors and the risk of coronary disease be utilized in planning preventive measures?

First, the studies identifying the contribution of sympathetically mediated cardiovascular responses to the risk of coronary disease must be carried out. Only a fraction of type A men between 40 and 50 years of age suffered a myocardial infarction during a 5-year observation period. If, for example, it could be shown that those type A men with a larger heart rate increase during sensory rejection behavior or a larger skeletal muscle vasoconstriction during sensory intake behavior are at greater risk to suffer a myocardial infarction than type A men with less intense cardiovascular responses, then an important intervening link between the type A factor and coronary disease would have been demonstrated. If clinical studies indicate a pathogenic role for such hyperresponsivity among type A individuals, the way would be clear to attempt to modify this intervening factor with the hope of preventing the onset of coronary disease. For example, biofeedback could be employed to train men with large heart rate increases during sensory rejection behavior to slow their heart rate during such behavior, or pharmacological means (such as the administration of propranolol) could be employed to achieve the same result. Similar efforts could be made to modify the physiological effects of sensory intake behavior if prospective studies indicate that these effects contribute to the risk of coronary disease. In addition to factors such as type A behavior that have already been shown to be associated with increased risk of coronary disease, the various measures of perceptual style that appear to be related to cardiovascular function could also enhance our ability to define further the risk of coronary disease.

Table 2 summarizes the variables and mechanisms that possibly mediate relationships between psychosocial factors and behavior, together with possible intervention strategies. These intervening mechanisms, although based on solid investigation, have yet to be shown as actually fulfilling such a role. Studies designed to test the validity of such mediational roles will undoubtedly add to our understanding of the nature of this empirical association. Moreover, it is through the identification of such intervening mechanisms that our efforts to prevent coronary disease will be most intelligently guided. Finally, understanding of the possible etiological role of psychosocial factors in coronary disease will be strengthened by a consideration of the potent intervening mechanisms that have been outlined in this chapter.

REFERENCES

1. Abrahams, V. C., Hilton, S. M., and Zbrozyna, A.: Active muscle vasodilatation produced by stimulation of the brain stem: its significance in the defense reaction, J. Physiol. **154:**491, 1960.
2. Abramson, D. I., and Ferris, E. B., Jr.: Response of blood vessels in the resting hand and forearm to various stimuli, Am. Heart J. **19:**541, 1941.
3. Adams, D. B., et al.: Relation of cardiovascular changes in fighting to emotion and exercise, J. Physiol. **212:**321, 1970.
4. Anderson, D. E., and Brady, J. V.: Preavoidance blood pressure elevations accompanied by heart rate decreases in the dog, Science **172:**595, 1971.
5. Anderson, D. E., and Tosheff, J. G.: Cardiac output and total peripheral resistance changes during preavoidance periods in the dog, J. Appl. Physiol. **34:**650, 1973.
6. Benson, H., et al.: Behaviorally induced hypertension in the squirrel monkey, Circ. Res. (suppl.) **27:**1, 1970.
7. Bittker, T. E., et al.: Cardiovascular and neurophysiologic correlates of sensory intake and rejection. II. Interview behavior. Psychophysiology **12:**434, 1975.
8. Blumenthal, J. A., et al.: Type A behavior pattern and coronary atherosclerosis, Circulation **58:**634, 1978.
9. Brod, J., et al.: Circulatory changes underlying blood pressure during acute emotional stress in normotensive and hypertensive subjects, Clin. Sci. **18:**269, 1959.
10. Craig, K. D., and Wood, K.: Autonomic components of observers' responses to pictures of homicide victims and nude females, J. Exp. Res. Personality **5:**304, 1971.
11. Dembyoski, T. M., MacDougall, J. M., and Shields, J. L.: Physiologic reactions to social challenge in persons evidencing the type A coronary-prone behavior pattern, J. Hum. Stress **3:**2, 1977.
12. Folkow, B., and Rubinstein, E. H.: Cardiovascular effects of acute and chronic stimulation of the hypothalamic defense area in the rat, Acta Physiol. Scand. **68:**48, 1966.
13. Forsyth, R. P., and Harris, R. E.: Circulatory changes during stressful stimuli in rhesus monkeys, Circ. Res. (suppl.) **27:**1, 1970.
14. Frankenhauser, M.: Experimental approaches to the study of human behavior as related to neuroendocrine functions. In Levi, L., editor: Society, stress and disease, London, 1971, Oxford University Press.
15. Freis, E. D.: Effectiveness of drug therapy in hypertension: present status, Circ. Res. (suppl.) **29:**11, 1971.
16. Friedman, M., Rosenman, R. H., and Carroll, V.: Changes in serum cholesterol and blood clotting time in men subjected to cyclic variation of occupational stress, Circulation **17:** 852, 1958.
17. Friedman, M., Byers, S. O., Diamant, J., et al.: Plasma catecholamine response of coronary-prone subjects (Type A) to a specific challenge, Metabolism **24:**205, 1975.
18. Goldstein, H. S., et al.: Psychological differentiation and specificity of response, J. Nerv. Ment. Dis. **151:**97, 1970.
19. Gunn, C. G., Friedman, M., and Byers, S. O.: Effect of chronic hypothalamic stimulation upon cholesterol-induced atherosclerosis in the rabbit, J. Clin. Invest. **39:**1963, 1960.
20. Gutstein, W. H., Lewis, L., and Schneck, D. J.: Plasma triglyceride rise in the rat following hypothalamic stimulation, Vasc. Dis. **4:**89, 1967.
21. Haft, J. I., et al.: Intravascular platelet aggregation in the heart induced by norepinephrine, Circulation **46:**698, 1972.
22. Harlan, W. R., Jr., et al.: Constitutional and environmental factors related to serum lipid and lipoprotein levels, Ann. Intern. Med. **66:**540, 1967.
23. Harris, R. E., and Singer, M. T.: The interaction of personality and stress in the pathogenesis of essential hypertension. In Hypertension: proceedings of the Council on High Blood Pressure Research, New York, 1967, American Heart Association.
24. Henry, J. P., Ely, D. L., and Stephens, P. M.: Mental factors and cardiovascular disease, Psychiatr. Ann. **2:**25, 1972.

25. Jones, R. J.: Atherosclerosis: proceedings of the second international symposium, New York, 1970, Springer-Verlag New York, Inc.
26. Keys, A.: The individual risk of coronary heart disease, Ann. N. Y. Acad. Sci. **134:**1046, 1966.
27. Keys, A.: Cardiology: the essentiality of prevention, Minn. Med. **52:**1191, 1969.
27a. Keys, A., Taylor, H. L., Blackburn, H., et al.: Mortality and coronary heart disease among men studied for 23 years, Arch. Intern. Med. **128:**201, 1971.
28. Lacey, J. I., et al.: The visceral level: situational determinants and behavioral correlates of autonomic response patterns. In Knopp, P. H., editor: Expression of the emotions in man, New York, 1963, International Universities Press.
29. Lamprecht, F., Williams, R. B., and Kopin, I. J.: Serum dopamine-beta-hydroxylase during development of immobilization—induced hypertension, Endocrinology **92:**953, 1973.
30. Lazarus, R. S.: Psychological stress and the coping process, New York, 1966, McGraw-Hill Book Co.
31. Manuck, S. B., Craft, S., and Gold, K. S.: Coronary-prone behavior pattern and cardiovascular response, Psychophysiol. **15:**403, 1978.
32. Mason, J. W.: A re-evaluation of the concept of non-specificity in stress theory, J. Psychiatr. Res. **8:**323, 1971.
33. McGough, W. E., Silverman, A. J., and Bogdonoff, M. D.: Patterns of fat mobilization in field-dependent and field-independent subjects, Psychosom. Med. **27:**245, 1965.
34. McKegney, F. P., and Williams, R. B.: Psychological aspects of hypertension. II. The differential influence of interview variables on blood pressure, Am. J. Psychiatr. **123:**1539, 1967.
35. Obrist, P. A., Lawler, J. E., and Gaebelein, C. J.: A psychobiological perspective on the cardiovascular system. In DiCara, L. V., editor: Advances in limbic and autonomic nervous system research, New York, 1973, Plenum Publishing Corp.
36. Raab, W.: Cardiotoxic biochemical effects of emotional-environmental stressors-fundamentals of psychocardiology. In Levi, L., editor: Society, stress and disease, London, 1971, Oxford University Press.
37. Raff, C. S., et al.: Paper presented at a meeting of the Southeastern Psychological Association, New Orleans, February, 1969.
38. Rahe, R. H., et al.: Group therapy in the outpatient management of post-myocardial infarction patients, Psychiatr. Med. **4:**77, 1973.
39. Rosenman, R. H., et al.: Coronary heart disease in the Western Collaborative Group Study: a follow-up experience of 4½ years, J. Chronic Dis. **23:**173, 1970.
40. Schechter, G., and Buchsbaum, M. S.: The effects of attention, stimulus intensity, and individual differences on the average evoked response, Psychophysiology **10:**392, 1973.
41. Silverman, A. J., and McGough, W. E.: Perceptual relationships to peripheral venous tone, J. Psychosom. Res. **15:**199, 1971.
42. Silverman, A. J., McGough, W. E., and Bogdonoff, M. D.: Perceptual correlates of the physiological response to insulin, Psychosom. Med. **29:**252, 1967.
43. Singer, M. T.: Enduring personality styles and responses to stress, Trans. Assoc. Life Ins. Med. Dir. Am. **51:**150, 1967.
44. Stead, E. A., Jr., et al.: The cardiac output in male subjects as measured by the technique of right atrial catheterization. Normal values with observations on the effect of anxiety and tilting, J. Clin. Invest. **24:**326, 1945.
45. Thomas, C. B.: The precursors of hypertension and coronary artery disease insights from studies of biological variation, Ann. N.Y. Acad. Sci. **134:**1028, 1966.
46. Weiner, H.: Some psychological factors related to cardiovascular responses: a logical and empirical analysis. In Roessler, R., and Greenfield, W. S., editors: Physiological correlates of psychological disorders, Madison, Wisc., 1962, University of Wisconsin Press.
47. Williams, R. B., and Eichelman, B.: Social setting; influence upon physiological response to electric shock in the rat, Science **174:**613, 1971.
48. Williams, R. B., Eichelman, B., and Ng, L. K. Y.: Patterns of sympathetic nervous system discharge and blood pressure response to foot shock in the rat, Psychophysiology **16:**89, 1978.
49. Williams, R. B., Ng, L. K. Y., and Eichelman, B.: Brain amine depletion reverses the blood response to foot shock in the rat, Nature (New Biol.) **240:**276, 1972.
50. Williams, R. B., Richardson, J. S., and

Eichelman, B. S.: Location of central nervous system neurones mediating blood pressure response of rats to shock-induced fighting, J. Behav. Med. **1**:177, 1978.

51. Williams, R. B., et al.: Peripheral sympathetic nerve activity and sensory intake behavior: a newly recognized association. Paper presented at the annual meeting of the American Psychosomatic Society, Philadelphia, 1974.
52. Williams, R. B., et al.: Cardiovascular and neurophysiologic correlates of sensory intake and rejection. I. Effect of cognitive tasks, Psychophysiology **12**:427, 1975.
53. Wolf, S.: Psychosocial forces in myocardial infarction and sudden death. In Levi, L., editor: Society, stress and disease, London, 1971, Oxford University Press.
54. Wyatt, R. J., et al.: Resting plasma catecholamine concentrations in patients with depression and anxiety, Arch. Gen. Psychiatr. **24**:65, 1971.

SECTION TWO

ACUTE CARE

4

Preadmission behavior

W. DOYLE GENTRY

One might expect individuals who experience symptoms of an acute myocardial infarction—chest pain, sweating, shortness of breath, and dizziness—to react quickly in seeking medical attention. Unfortunately, this is often not the case. Approximately 50% of all patients who die suddenly after experiencing symptoms of myocardial infarction do so within 1 hour after onset of symptoms and prior to receiving any type of medical assistance. The majority (70%) of such deaths, in fact, occur within 15 minutes after the individual experiences hard symptoms of infarction.[4] Medically, deaths resulting from myocardial infarction that occur before a patient reaches a hospital appear to be the result of ventricular fibrillation associated with the early phases of infarction, a condition that is potentially reversible. Psychologically, such deaths appear to be the result of faulty symptom attribution and unnecessary delay on the part of the person experiencing the myocardial infarction.

THE TYPICAL RESPONSE

The typical response of actual or potential coronary patients during the period prior to hospital admission is to delay seeking medical advice or treatment far beyond the critical 1-hour period associated with sudden death. As shown in Fig. 5, the hospital arrival time for such patients can range from less than 1 hour up to several days.[7] About 56% of coronary patients arrive at the hospital in less than 4 hours, 28% take from 4 to 14 hours, and 16% arrive after more than 14 hours. The median time for hospital arrival is between 2½ and 4 hours after the onset of symptoms.[4,6,10,11]

Approximately 65% of the time between symptom onset and arrival at the hospital involves what has been referred to as the patient's *decision time,* that is, the interval between the onset of acute coronary symptoms and the patient's decision to get medical help. It is on this segment of time that investigators have focused their attention in attempting to understand why patients delay seeking medical attention, and it is on this interval that much of the remaining discussion

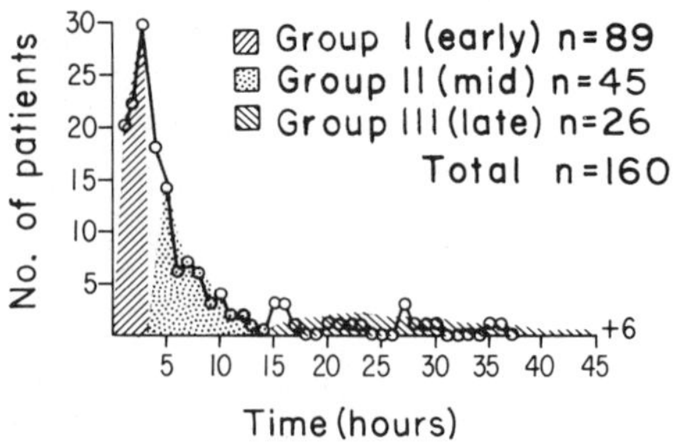

Fig. 5. Time taken by sample group of coronary patients in seeking medical assistance. Time is measured from onset of symptoms to arrival at a hospital. (From Moss, A. J., and Goldstein, S.: Circulation **41:**737, 1970.)

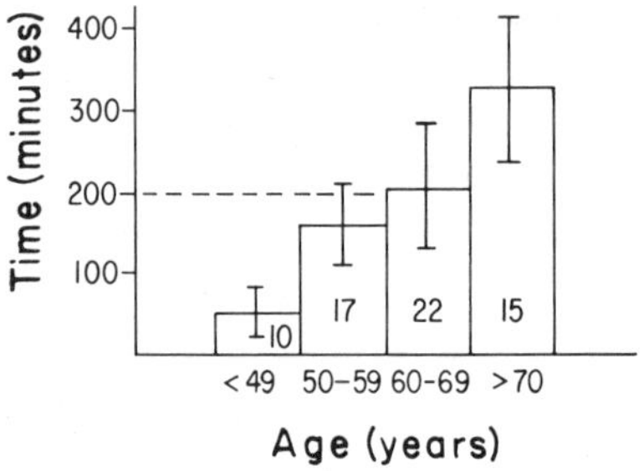

Fig. 6. Relationship between age of coronary patient and tendency to delay in seeking medical care. Time refers to patient's decision time. (From Moss, A. J., et al.: Am. J. Cardiol. **24:**659, 1969.)

will center. Another 25% of the time between onset and arrival at a hospital is essentially *unaccounted for;* Moss et al.[8] regard this as time for "human factors." This represents the time used by the patient and his family to contact a physician or ambulance, for the physician to render advice, and for all concerned to prepare themselves for going to the hospital. The final 10% of the time required for arrival at a hospital involves the actual *transportation time,* whether the patient travels by ambulance or car.

Coronary patients typically also fail to correctly relate their initial symptoms to a cardiac problem. Tjoe and Luria[12] report that only 21 of 75 patients admitted to a coronary care unit initially attributed their symptoms to a cardiac condition (Table 3). A much greater percentage of these patients attributed their symptoms to such causes as gallbladder disease, a cold, emphysema, diabetes, gas pains, and ulcers. In an earlier study, Olin and Hackett[9] similarly noted that only 10 of 32 patients with acute myocardial infarctions correctly diagnosed their conditions.

Table 3. Initial interpretation of symptoms by patients admitted to the cardiac care unit*

Symptom interpretation	Number of patients	Patients with past history of myocardial infarction	Patients without history of myocardial infarction
Heart problem	21	14	7
Gas, pain, ulcer	32	5	27
"Didn't know"	15	0	15
Others†	7	2	5
TOTAL	75	21	54

*From Tjoe, S. L., and Luria, M. H.: Chest **61**:617, 1972.
†Excessive smoking, gallbladder disease, cold, emphysema, and diabetes.

Fourteen of their patients explained their chest pain as resulting from indigestion, and seven more thought they were coming down with lung disease. In the two studies combined, 70% of the patients misinterpreted the cause of their symptoms.

FACTORS DETERMINING PREADMISSION BEHAVIOR

The factors determining a patient's preadmission behavior following an acute myocardial infarction fall into four categories: (1) demographic characteristics, (2) history of coronary disease, (3) the patient's perception of illness, and (4) the social context in which the onset of symptoms occurs.

Demographic characteristics

Three studies[1,7,8] have indicated a significant relationship between *age* and the time taken by coronary patients to arrive at a hospital; older patients take considerably more time to seek medical help than younger patients. This relationship is shown in Fig. 6. *Sex* has also been related to delay, with men manifesting a shorter decision time than women. *Educational background, marital status, occupation, ethnicity, religious affiliation,* and *socioeconomic class,* on the other hand, appear to have no relationship to preadmission behavior.

History of coronary disease

Another characteristic important in determining preadmission behavior is the patient's *history of coronary disease.* As noted in Table 3, patients with a past history of myocardial infarction were consistently better able to diagnose their initial symptoms as cardiac problems than were patients without a history of myocardial infarction. Sixty-seven percent of the former group were able to correctly identify their coronary symptoms, as compared with only 13% of the latter group. However, with respect to delay in seeking medical assistance, a history of coronary disease for the most part seems either to have no effect[4] or may in fact increase the time required for a patient to seek proper care. Alonzo,[1] for example, has noted that patients with a history of coronary disease and/or other chronic diseases tend to become involved in circuitous care-seeking behavior, whereas patients with little or no evidence of chronic disease tend to follow an expedient and direct path to the hospital. Goldstein et al.[5] also found that patients with a history of peptic ulcer disease and hypertension tended to evidence a much shorter decision time and arrived at a hospital more quickly than patients with a history of angina, diabetes, and myocardial infarction.

Perception of illness

Moss et al.[8] have emphasized that there are three separate cognitive functions required in making a decision to seek medical help following the onset of symptoms: (1) *perception* of the presenting symptoms, (2) *recognition* of the meaning and seriousness of the symptoms, and (3) *realization* that medical care is indicated for the treatment of such symptoms. To the extent that a patient follows this cognitive sequence of perception-recognition-realization, he should arrive at the proper medical facility, whether physician's office, emergency room, or coronary care unit, in a reasonably short time; to the extent that he is unable to follow the sequence, he will delay in seeking care.

Olin and Hackett[9] have noted that all patients admitted to the coronary care unit had experienced some symptoms, primarily acute chest pain, during the preadmission phase of their illness. However, they also noted that the majority attributed their symptoms to other causes. In a related study, Hackett and Cassem[6] found a significant relationship between symptom attribution and delay in seeking medical treatment; patients who recognized that they had something wrong with their heart sought help sooner than those who displaced the cause of their symptoms to other organ systems. Hackett and Cassem[6] further observed that delay in arriving at a hospital was in part a function of the patient's subjective appraisal of the severity of his symptoms prior to coming in; patients who believed their symptoms to be severe sought help more quickly than patients who believed their symptoms were less severe. Similarly, Alonzo[1] has indicated that coronary patients seek care more directly when they experience their symptoms as "noxious" and "uncontrollable," as opposed to "less noxious" and "manageable." Gentry and Haney[3] reported that coronary patients who acknowledged a greater degree of perceived illness tended to delay less in getting to the hospital from the time of symptom onset than did patients who failed to see themselves as being ill.

Hackett and Cassem[6] and Olin and Hackett[9] have stressed the role of *denial* in altering the patient's recognition of the seriousness of his symptoms prior to seeking proper medical care. Denial is an adaptive psychological defense mechanism employed by the individual, consciously or unconsciously, to alleviate anxiety and apprehension generated by the possibilities of imminent death and/or helplessness. To illustrate the use of denial in a patient newly admitted to a coronary care unit, Olin and Hackett[9] cite the following case:

> A 65-year-old medical technician had sustained a previous myocardial infarction ten years before his present admission. At that time he had experienced severe precordial pain which he attributed to indigestion. After being given morphine at home in preparation for the trip to the hospital, he started to dress for work because he felt so much better. He finally consented to hospitalization only because he "liked the doctors so much." In the current episode he again diagnosed his condition as stomach trouble and waited five hours before calling a doctor. He made the call only when the pain became unbearable. After being told the diagnosis, he felt as though his life was ended and spoke of suicide, but did not attempt it.*

While denial may serve a useful purpose in momentarily reducing an unpleasant affect (anxiety or depression) in the coronary patient, it may also serve to reduce long-term chances for proper medical care and thus survival. As Hackett and Cassem[6] note, denial is related to symptom displacement and the influence of another person on the decision to seek help. Patients operating under "minimal denial" more often recognized their heart as the source of the trouble and generally did not require the assistance of others around them—spouse and family—in making the decision to seek medical advice. This is in contrast to the response of patients characterized by "maximal denial," who believed their trouble was caused by other organ systems and tended to put off consulting a physician until others urged them to do so. Gentry and Haney[3] also observed that patients reporting high levels of concern about death tended to delay less in getting to the hospital than patients with similar symptoms who were less concerned about dying.

Finally, the presence of prodromal symptoms can contribute to an unnecessary and dangerous delay in seeking medical care. Both Moss and Goldstein[7] and Goldstein et al.[5] found that patients with a previous history of angina and/or prodromal symptoms prior to the onset of such acute symptoms tended to delay in getting help; in their words, such patients may simply have difficulty in distinguishing "the same old symptoms from something new and different."

Social context

Alonzo[1] notes that most investigators of the preadmission behavior of coronary patients have employed a model of "psychological individualism" that ignores the social context in which the patient finds himself at the time of symptom onset. Thus behaviors that Hackett and Cassem[6] and Olin and Hackett[9] might see as evidence of denial constitute for Alonzo the "social reality with which ill individuals must cope."[1] For example, several investigators have found that the *time of*

*From Olin, H. L., and Hackett, T. P.: The denial of chest pain in 32 patients with acute myocardial infarction, J.A.M.A. **190:**977, 1964.

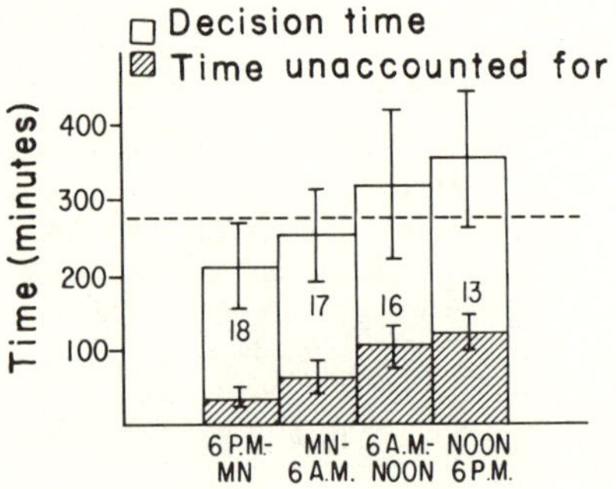

Fig. 7. Relationship between time of day of onset of acute coronary symptoms and patients' decision time and time unaccounted for. (From Moss, A. J., et al.: Am. J. Cardiol. **24:**659, 1969.)

day and *day of the week* on which acute symptoms occur in part determine the patient's pattern of preadmission behavior.[7,8,12] As shown in Figs. 7 and 8, the greatest delays in seeking medical attention occurred when patients experienced the onset of symptoms during the day and on weekends. Goldstein et al.[5] also noted a significant shortening of delay in patients whose symptoms occurred during working as opposed to off-work hours. Alonzo[1] and Goldstein et al.[5] found too that there was less delay if patients experienced the onset of symptoms when others, particularly spouses, were present.

The decision time and eventual amount of time required for patients to arrive at a hospital, of course, are shorter when the patient makes the decision to seek medical advice or treatment himself. This fact is borne out in studies by Moss et al.,[8] Moss and Goldstein,[7] and Alonzo.[1] Gentry and Haney[3] have noted that patients admitted to a coronary care unit tend to make the decision to seek medical attention themselves when they believe they have sustained a heart attack.

SELF-TREATMENT AND NONTHERAPEUTIC ACTIVITIES

Part of the preadmission behavior manifested by patients involves self-treatment and nontherapeutic activities[4,10,11] that serve to prolong the time before hospitalization. Simon et al.[11] have noted that patients who used previously prescribed medications (nitroglycerin, cardiac glycosides, or antihypertensive drugs) following the onset of symptoms took significantly longer to get to the hospital than patients who did not have such drugs on hand. A similar relationship was found between delay and the use of patient medications; only 10% of the patients who arrived at a hospital in less than 1 hour used such medicines as compared with 41% of the patients who arrived after more than 12 hours. Similarly, patients

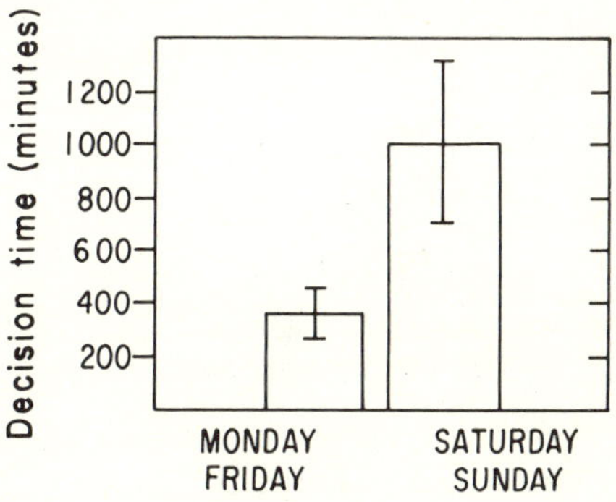

Fig. 8. Decision time related to day of symptom onset for coronary patients. (From Tjoe, S. L., and Luria, M. H.: Chest **61:**617, 1972.)

who were able to modify existing social obligations and who did not have to become involved in extensive "washing-up and changing clothes" behaviors delayed less in getting proper care than did those who were compelled to carry out such nontherapeutic activities. As Simon et al.[11] point out, "How one utilizes time as a resource is therefore a major determinant of whether one dies outside the hospital setting or is hospitalized."

The following dialogue from a clinical interview with a 39-year-old male patient recuperating from a myocardial infarction illustrates the interplay between denial, symptom attribution, presence of the spouse, decision making, self-treatment, and delay in seeking medical assistance:[2]

Dr.: Can you tell me about what brought you to the hospital? Did you have a heart attack?
Pt.: Well, when they brought me in, they said I was having one. To me, it was just chest pain, something like indigestion.
Dr.: How long was it between the time you felt the chest pain and the time you got to the hospital?
Pt.: Probably an hour to an hour and a half. At first the pain wasn't as severe as it was (later on)—just a pain, not too severe then.
Dr.: Were you by yourself when you experienced this chest pain?
Pt.: No, my wife had just come home from work.
Dr.: Did you make the decision to come to the hospital? Did you talk this over with her? Or did she make the decision?
Pt.: Well, I was trying to get something to help the indigestion. I told her where the pain was and she told me where some Maalox was and I thought I'd try it. I tried it and it didn't work, and she took a quick look at me and saw I was sweating and still had the pain. She decided that I needed to come to the hospital right then. But by then I was in a lot of pain.
Dr.: Did you, by the time you got to the hospital with the increased pain, begin to think that this might be something more than just indigestion?
Pt.: Well, she had just told me, as we left the house, that she thought I probably was having a heart attack. . . .

It is clear that this patient, who still failed to accept the reality of myocardial infarction even after receiving cardiac catheterization and spending several days in the coronary care unit, had minimized the severity of his chest pain at initial onset and had further misattributed the cause of the pain to indigestion, thus delaying any attempt at seeking medical consultation and/or assistance. His denial of the true nature of his symptoms, more importantly, had caused him to depend totally on his wife to correctly diagnose the cause of his symptoms, decide that hospitalization was essential, and actually transport him to the medical facility. She was the one who had properly worked through the perception-recognition-realization sequence necessary for adaptive preadmission behavior, not the patient. Had she not arrived home at the time the patient was beginning to experience the hard symptoms of acute infarction, it is highly probable that he would have continued to look for noncardiac causes for his pain and discomfort, to engage in even more attempts at self-treatment, and thus increase the delay in seeking proper medical care. The result could well have been sudden cardiac death.

PHYSICIAN DELAY

The effect of consultation with a physician on the patient's decision time and time elapsed before arrival at a hospital has also been examined. As shown in Table 4, about 26% of the patients studied by Simon et al.[11] did not consult a physician prior to arriving at a hospital. Of the remaining patients who did seek consultation, 71% were involved with the physician for less than 1 hour and thus were not significantly delayed in getting to the hospital; the remaining 29% of these patients, however, were involved with a physician for several hours and thus took much longer to eventually get proper hospital care. Simon et al.[11] have found that such long delays usually resulted from the patient's having to make an office call to the physician in question or wait for the physician to visit his home.

With respect to physician delay, Tjoe and Luria[12] have observed:

> Further analysis of delay indicates that the second most important cause can be attributed to physicians. Physicians delay time may account for as much as two or three days or longer. In most cases it appears due to diagnostic uncertainty. . . . Less delay in patient evaluation together with earlier hospitalization might help reduce coronary disease mortality.*

Hackett and Cassem[6] are perhaps the strongest in their criticism of physician delay regarding coronary patients. For the 12 patients out of 100 that were delayed by physician consultation in getting to the hospital, these authors observed:

> The physician employed the same maneuvers used by patients who delayed. He either blamed other organ systems or minimized the pain by calling it angina. In some cases, medication was given and the patient was instructed to wait. In other cases, an appointment

*From Tjoe, S. L., and Luria, M. H.: Delays in reaching the cardiac care unit: an analysis, Chest **61:**617, 1972.

Table 4. Distribution of medical decision time: the time taken by the physician to reach a decision to hospitalize the patient*

Time	Number of patients†	Percent‡	Cumulative percent
Physician consultation	(42)	(26.2)	
Minutes			
≤15	49	41.5	41.5
16-30	8	6.8	48.3
31-60	14	11.8	60.1
Hours			
1-2	13	11.0	71.1
2-3	8	6.8	77.9
3-6	8	6.8	84.7
6-12	4	3.4	88.1
>12	14	11.9	100.0
TOTAL	160		

*Modified from Simon, A. B., et al.: Am. J. Cardiol. **30**:476, 1972.
†In 42 instances (26.2%) no physician was contacted prior to the patient's arrival at the hospital.
‡Percent is expressed as percent of those consulting a physician before reaching the hospital.

> was made for an office visit the next day. . . . One of the delaying doctors later admitted that he thought his patient was simply exaggerating his pain. In fact, this same physician doubted that the patient had true coronary disease until it was amply demonstrated angiographically.*

They concluded that since referral to a hospital is a simple matter, no adequate explanation can be given for the procrastination of a physician, which leads obviously to reduced chances of survival for his patients.

Alonzo[1] found that individuals who followed an expedient and direct path to the hospital after experiencing the onset of symptoms typically recognized emergency room evaluation as a more direct source of care than physician consultation or received medical consultation from a general practitioner. Those patients who were involved in more circuitous care-seeking behavior and who thus delayed their arrival at the hospital generally either had an established, deferential relationship with their physician or had consulted an internist or cardiologist. The amount of time required for patient evaluation prior to hospitalization also varied greatly among physicians. Physicians evaluated and referred older patients quickly and took more time to evaluate younger, less diseased individuals. Similarly, where the physician had a long-standing relationship with the patient, evaluation and referral proceeded quickly; where the physician did not know the patient or had only minimal, episodic contact with him, evaluation was prolonged.

*Hackett, T. P., and Cassem, N. H.: Factors contributing to delay in responding to the signs and symptoms of acute myocardial infarction, Am. J. Cardiol. **24**:651, 1969.

PREADMISSION BEHAVIOR AND MORTALITY

It was pointed out at the beginning of this discussion that many patients who die suddenly from acute myocardial infarction do so within 1 hour after the onset of symptoms. Obviously any unnecessary delay or indecision on the patient's part, not to mention that of the physician and others, greatly reduces the patient's chances of survival. In fact, even if the patient reaches the hospital alive, the delay involved in his getting there may affect his chances for a successful recovery. Moss and Goldstein[7] have noted that only 10% of "early arrivals" died in the hospital as compared with 27% of the "late arrivals," a mortality rate almost three times as great. Whether this increased mortality is a result solely of delay in getting to the hospital is not clear, as the "early arrivals" were younger as a group than the "late arrivals" and also had less history of angina and diabetes. However, whether independent of other factors or not, delay is still a critical variable in determining the coronary patient's prognosis for recovery subsequent to myocardial infarction.

SUMMARY

The preceding description of preadmission behavior of individuals experiencing symptoms of an acute myocardial infarction and the factors that appear to determine such behavior suggests several conclusions. First, it seems clear that the burden of responsibility for seeking proper medical attention after symptom onset does not rest solely with the patient. Others who are not medical professionals, especially spouse and family, as well as physicians contacted prior to hospitalization can play a vital role in helping the patient to decide that such symptoms are indeed serious and warrant medical care. Second, it is not any single characteristic of an individual patient (age, sex, history of coronary disease, or use of psychological defense mechanisms such as denial) that wholly determines whether and when the patient seeks help, but rather all of these factors and more. Perhaps most important is the social context in which the patient finds himself at the time of symptom onset. If there are others around to help him decide in favor of seeking medical advice and treatment, if he is not involved in ongoing social functions that would be difficult to interrupt, or if the symptoms first occur during a time of day and day of the week when they seem more serious (during the middle of the night), the patient will generally respond more quickly in getting to a hospital or to some other type of medical care facility. If the conditions are different, if he is alone watching television during the day on Saturday, for example, he may be unable to decide what to make of the symptoms, delay, and thus die before ever receiving the care that could save his life.

Finally, one might ask what could be done to change this typical pattern of behavior in coronary patients to reduce unnecessary mortality prior to hospitalization or death that results from delay in getting proper care. Our answer to this is simple—education. Patients must be educated to recognize the symptoms of myocardial infarction, those that appear both in the prodromal period and in the acute phase. They must be taught, for example, that chest pain is by far the most common symptom of infarction and thus they should not be falsely reassured by the fact that they have not as yet experienced any respiratory symptoms (shortness of breath). If they have a history of angina or other chronic disease, they must be made aware of the fact that such conditions often contribute to unnecessary delay and thus a poorer prognosis for survival—whether or not they can distinguish "something new from the same old thing" they should seek medical advice. Physicians too must be educated. They must be told that physician delay appears to be the second most important cause of patients not securing help in time and that office visits or house calls at such a time may be life-threatening to their patients.

REFERENCES

1. Alonzo, A. A.: Illness behavior during acute episodes of coronary heart disease, Unpublished Ph.D. thesis, University of California, Berkeley, 1973.
2. Gentry, W. D.: Pre-hospital behavior, Psychiatr. Ann. In press.
3. Gentry, W. D., and Haney, T.: Emotional and behavioral reaction to acute myocardial infarction, Heart Lung **4:**738, 1975.
4. Gillum, R. F., et al.: Delay in the prehospital phase of acute myocardial infarction, Arch. Intern. Med. **136:**649, 1976.
5. Goldstein, S., Moss, A. J., and Greene, W.: Sudden death in acute myocardial infarction, Arch. Intern. Med. **129:**720, 1972.
6. Hackett, T. P., and Cassem, N. H.: Factors contributing to delay in responding to the signs and symptoms of acute myocardial infarction, Am. J. Cardiol. **24:**651, 1969.
7. Moss, A. J., and Goldstein, S.: The prehospital phase of acute myocardial infarction, Circulation **41:**737, 1970.
8. Moss, A. J., Wynar, B., and Goldstein, S.: Delay in hospitalization during the acute coronary period, Am. J. Cardiol. **24:**659, 1969.
9. Olin, H. S., and Hackett, T. P.: The denial of chest pain in 32 patients with acute myocardial infarction, J.A.M.A. **190:**977, 1964.
10. Simon, A. B., Alonzo, A. A., and Feinleib, M.: Patient response to acute episodes of coronary heart disease, Arch. Intern. Med. **133:** 824, 1974.
11. Simon, A. B., Feinleib, M., and Thompson, H. K.: Components of delay in the prehospital phase of acute myocardial infarction, Am. J. Cardiol. **30:**476, 1972.
12. Tjoe, S. L., and Luria, M. H.: Delays in reaching the cardiac care unit: an analysis, Chest **61:**617, 1972.

5

Human contact, coping, and cardiac function in coronary patients

SUE ANN THOMAS
JAMES J. LYNCH

Coronary care units (CCUs), the patients in them, and the staff who treat these patients present complex and divergent sets of physical and psychodynamic variables. Therefore, any description of the interaction of coping mechanisms, human contact, and physiological functioning within this acute hospital setting is complicated. In these units, however, the difference between life and death is often based on immediate clinical judgments and technical procedures, and complexities are viewed as something that ought to be kept to the bare minimum. The dominant set is to base all clinical judgments on observable pathology and to reduce all clinical procedures into a system in which each action has measurable consequences.

Does patient survival in coronary care units really hinge on coming to grips with complex psychological issues? Do the two somewhat different conceptual frameworks, the psychological and the physiological orientation, really mix? Can one really pay attention to the physical well-being of a patient and at the same time pay more than lip service to the complex psychological makeup of the patient and staff?

There is curiously a temptation to answer these important questions quite glibly in the affirmative by asserting unequivocally that attending to psychological variables makes a difference. After all, numerous cases can be cited in which neglect of psychological aspects precipitated sudden death.[15] Even the most ordinary forms of human contact can alter the ongoing frequency of arrhythmias in coronary care patients.* Such evidence, however, must be weighed by the clinician along with the physiological factors that influence the incidence of arrhythmias.

*See Lynch, et al.[16,18,19] Mills, et al.[21] and Thomas et al.[23]

One is immediately struck by the sharp contrast between the description and prescription of advice to be given in the topic of "things psychological" and the precision of other aspects of clinical care within a coronary care unit. In life-and-death situations, the neat, precise regulation of xylocaine to the milligram per kilogram of body weight and the occurrence of premature ventricular contractions gives this prescriptive advice immediate relevance. Or view the precision involved in reading and interpreting the electrocardiogram and sense the utility and power such information carries with it. The overriding concern in units charged with life and death decisions is, in fact, nakedly pragmatic. Does the information work and how immediately useful is it? Therein lies a central problem that is at best highly complex and at worst perhaps irresolvable. For clearly the cardiovascular system is a pump that obeys precise hemodynamic principles that can be readily measured.

Even the most radically mechanistic physician or nurse, however, knows that the hemodynamic pump they are treating resides within a human being who seems to be far more than a machine. There is virtually no cardiologist or coronary care unit nurse who would state that psychological factors are not important in coronary care, in cardiac functioning, and indeed in long-term survival. That these factors are important seems both empirically and intuitively obvious. Yet if you ask many of these same clinicians how they approach the treatment of psychological problems of patients in coronary care units, they often will become slightly irritated, ask you to implicitly agree that the whole problem is too complicated, or point toward their use of antianxiety agents. If a coronary patient becomes blatantly psychotic, obviously depressed, or openly anxious, they will add that a psychiatrist can be called in for a consultation. Beyond these global approaches, psychological problems are often viewed as being so complicated or vague that many believe there is little anyone can do about them. This represents what has been called a widespread, shared feeling of therapeutic nihilism.[15]

The mechanistic point of view is easy to criticize, but it does contain a certain element of intellectual honesty that deserves to be recognized. All too often the clinicians who assert the opposite point of view—that psychological mechanisms ought to be attended to in coronary patients—also maintain a point of view that borders on self-deception. Some of the psychologically minded clinicians tend to focus exclusively on coronary patients during the brief period of hospitalization. They outline elegant strategies for identifying maladaptive coping mechanisms in patients during this phase of critical care. They provide clear-cut and precise descriptions of depression, denial mechanisms, defensive patterns, and anxiety reactions in coronary patients and even outlines of clinical ways to approach these problems. The importance of these observations should not be minimized, for the evidence strongly suggests that emotional state can alter neurophysiological and neuroendocrine functioning and thus directly influence coronary functioning after a myocardial infarction.[11,13,20,24] What is needed, however, is a closer examination of the entire context in which these psychological assessments are made. Unfortunately, the larger sociocultural existence of these patients is usually ignored. Some clinicians believe that by attending to the psychological status of coronary patients they have "treated" the whole person. They believe that a patient's depression or anxiety can be treated in the coronary care unit, while at the same time the social and economic conditions that first brought many of these patients to such units are ignored. Patients who are lonely, isolated, and impoverished are led to implicitly believe that their depression or denial is largely a result of their "heart attack" and can be solved as their physiological problems are resolved. Clearly, a balance must be found between those persons who believe the whole topic of psychological coping mechanisms is too complicated and therefore best ignored and those persons who claim that such mechanisms can be diagnosed and treated in coronary patients, while the larger realities of these patients' existences are ignored.

Within the context of the coronary care unit, it is important to emphasize that many hospital personnel are already doing an excellent job comforting and supporting patients and they often do it with virtually no formal training in psychology or psychiatry. They very beautifully fulfill Sir William Osler's prescriptive advice that the best way to care for a patient is to simply care about the patient. But as knowledge has grown, it has tended to become more specialized. Many coronary care unit personnel who are superbly trained in cardiovascular hemodynamics are now left with the feeling that there is this other scientific field, psychiatry and psychology, that has an equally vast amount of technical knowledge about which they know very little. Given an awareness that they know so little about psychology, they are implicitly made to believe that they best stay away from things psychological in their patients and leave this domain to other "experts." As knowledge becomes specialized and fragmented, all too often the unfortunate victims are the patients, whose treatment also becomes fragmented in the process. Often issues of human compassion and human concern have been obscured by a barrage of psychological jargon that leads coronary care unit personnel to deed over even elementary human concerns to psychologists or psychiatrists who are viewed as "experts" in the area.

While re-emphasizing that a patient's stay in a coronary care unit is but a small segment of a patient's life span and that psychological coping is a process that extends both prior to and hopefully long after a patient's brief period of hospitalization, nevertheless, there are important aspects of this critical period that merit close examination. Such an examination involves at least three different perspectives: (1) the structure and location of the coronary care units in hospitals, (2) the staff, and (3) the patients. Even though these three components obviously interact and are woven together, it may be helpful to examine them separately.

CORONARY CARE UNITS

It is important to emphasize that coronary care units, as specialized units within hospitals, are a relatively recent evolutionary development, having gradually become separate hospital entities over the past two decades. With advancing electronic technology, it became possible to continuously monitor the heart rhythm of patients. Along with this development, procedures were standardized to maintain a continuous intravenous drip, allowing the staff to give medications to suppress cardiac arrhythmias, stimulate heart rate, or alter blood pressure without delay. Perhaps the most important development was the introduction of specialized training courses given not only to internists and cardiologists but to all the medical staff including resident physicians and nurses that enabled them to recognize cardiac complications early and to treat them aggressively.

Because these units have gradually evolved, most hospital personnel have been able to adapt to the new technology and the new types of units. Patients, however, may not have been a patient in a hospital since their birth, and for them these units appear very strange, sometimes totally overwhelming. The psychological impact of suddenly being whisked into a coronary care unit, intravenous needles in one's arms, tubes in one's nose, electrodes on one's chest recording every heartbeat on television monitors and threatened with possible imminent death has been described by patients as psychologically shattering.[14] While the staff of coronary units has become acclimated to these new environments, they tend to forget how very strange and threatening these units appear to many patients. Clearly some explanation of EKG sensors and the heart monitor itself is necessary.

Beyond these elementary explanations, however, looms a far more perplexing problem, that of nonverbal communications embedded in the structure of a coronary care unit itself. Research on the social psychology of psychological experiments has revealed that the most significant communication between a research investigator and a subject does not involve words at all, but is instead couched in the context and structure within which the communication occurs.[22] To a large extent, structural communications implicitly control the behavior of everyone who enters these units, whether they are staff, patients, or visitors. For example, the staff need not tell a patient that he or she is dependent on them for survival, the entire context of the unit is one that demands total dependency. Such dependency, in turn, often engenders regressive behavior patterns in patients. Patients who are placed in dependent roles seem to need to feel they are being cared for and closely watched by a competent staff. The need for being cared for by competent clinicians sometimes appears in surprising ways that involve the very structure of coronary care units. These units can vary from 12- to 15-bed open units to private or semiprivate rooms. A number of reports have alluded to the disturbing nature of these environments,[8] including the effects such units have on the disturbance of sleep.[3,12] The open units would seem, on first analysis, to be far more anxiety provoking. The patients can see one another, they are disturbed frequently by a variety of environmental crises, and they may even witness another patient's cardiac arrest. It has been argued, for example, by Broughton and Baron[1] that the noisy, active environment of an open coronary unit contributes to the serious sleep disturbance routinely seen in coronary patients. On the other hand, Hackett et al.[9] have argued that the type of unit is far less important than the psychological state of the individual patient.

In an attempt to answer the question as to the relative importance of having an open unit versus a semiprivate environment, we monitored the sleep patterns of a large number of patients in both environments.[4] The patients in the semiprivate rooms were all judged clinically to be less seriously ill and in less danger of suffering a cardiac arrest. The typical patient woke up at least thirteen times during the night, a rate of awakening far in excess of what one would normally expect. We observed, however, similar sleep disturbance in both the open unit and the semiprivate unit. This lack of consistent difference in measure of sleep disturbance between the two types of units is surprising for several reasons. The patients in the semiprivate rooms were judged to be more stable and in less danger of cardiac complications, thus requiring less immediate attention. Furthermore, few patients in semiprivate rooms had intravenous drips and movement was less confined. Finally, the patients in the open unit were exposed to far more environmental disturbances, all of which would seem to dispose the patients in semiprivate rooms to less disturbed sleep. Yet such was not the case. One way to interpret these findings is that patients in semiprivate rooms are not reassured by the constant presence of ward staff. Hence they have as great a difficulty sleeping as those in an open unit.

Some have argued that the therapeutic benefits of coronary care units must be weighed against the structural communications of threat and disruptive anxiety these units engender. The pros and cons of this debate are being heatedly argued now in the scientific community, and it appears that given the multidimensional character of the debate and the complexity of the issues involved, empirically conclusive answers will not be forthcoming for some time. In the meantime, the staffs of coronary care units are still responsible for the patients' well-being, both during their hospitalization and, implicitly, long after the patient leaves the hospital. The best that can be hoped for until more data are gathered is that the staff become sensitive to the nonverbal structural control that these units exercise over the patients' lives.

Coronary care unit staff

One of the more intriguing aspects of the scientific literature dealing with psychological processes in coronary care units is the almost exclusive focus on patients' coping mechanisms within these environments, leading one to suspect that the ability of the clinical staff to cope psychologically is more or less taken for granted. This stance is particularly intriguing in view of the time-honored psychodynamic formulations of psychoanalytically oriented therapy that suggest that all interactions between a patient and a therapist involve psychodynamic needs of both. Stated another way, a patient can only express those feelings and thoughts that the clinician is able to hear. While feelings of anxiety within the patient can keep him from expressing certain feelings, anxiety within the listener can also block expression of those same thoughts.[7] While it seems clear that the staff may have neither the time nor the inclination to engage in in-depth psychology or extensive analytical introspection, it must be recognized that the personalities of the staff do influence their ability to diagnose psychological struggles in their patients. Major variables such as the age, sex, and race of the patients and the staff enter into these situations. Does the relatively young age of some coronary unit nurses and physicians influence the psychological assessment of anxiety in elderly patients? A number of studies in other clinical areas have convincingly documented that these variables often intrude on the assessment of a patient's psychological status.[6]

Beyond these psychodynamic formulations, there are structural situations that deserve closer scrutiny. One is the compartmentalization of the treatment process. In many coronary care units, physicians and nurses deal in a most intense life-and-death struggle with human beings who are totally dependent on them. Yet often these professionals personally know virtually nothing of these patients' lives beyond the confines of the units. This is most glaring in large hospital settings in which the contact within the unit is most intense. A patient then is released sometimes never to be seen by that staff again. Klein et al.[13] have already shown the impact of these relationships on the cardiovascular status of coronary patients during hospitalization. They studied fourteen patients who were transferred from a coronary care unit to a general medical ward. Seven were moved abruptly without advance warning and without having the coronary unit staff visit them after transfer. Of these seven patients, five suffered recurrent cardiovascular complications while still in the hospital. They complained of being lonely, depressed, and feeling abandoned by the coronary unit staff. The other seven patients to be transferred out of the same unit were then followed by the coronary unit staff during the remainder of their stay in the hospital. While these patients also reported various emotional reactions to the transfer, none had recurrent cardiac complications.

Extraordinarily intense human relationships are made in coronary care units and then broken, forcing one to wonder whether the observations of Klein et al.[13] might have any carry-over implications to the patient's home. Intense relationships are demanded with people, some of whom will not live out the week. Many who do survive are then returned home to relatively isolated environments. Some patients go home to environments of such acute social isolation that they cannot even list one person who should be called in an emergency.[15] We have been following 220 randomly selected patients on a monthly basis after their release from the coronary care unit to assess the relative impact of physiological and psychosocial variables on long-term survival. Almost 50% of these patients were either single, widowed, or divorced. For many of these patients, the care and attention they received while in the hospital was in sharp contrast to the loneliness and isolation of their total lives. Yet it appears that the very structure of these units demand that the staff keep busy, allowing them to "overlook" the pathetic condition of many patients' lives and avoid thinking about the relationships they are ending every week.[2]

Supervisors of coronary care units should employ only those persons who are psychologically capable of working in them, or the pressures of working in these units will gradually take their toll. Gentry et al.,[5] for example, have looked at certain psychological characteristics of nurses working in coronary care units and found that they tended to score higher on indices of depression, hostility, and anxiety than nurses who worked in general medical wards. They suggest that this stems, at least in part, from overwhelming work loads, too much responsibility, cramped working space, poor doctor-nurse communications, and inadequate programs for continuing education.

And even while the structure quite clearly communicates to the patient its life-threatening nature, coronary care unit staffs often defend themselves from this anxiety and thus do not share their patients' concerns. For example, the staff can rather easily move in to support a patient's denial by the very process of diagnosing a myocardial infarction. Enzyme levels and EKGs give the conclusive answer, but that may take several days to confirm. Until the staff is certain, why not deny? By the time the staff knows for certain, unless complications develop, the patients are ready for transfer. If complications develop again, it is "wait and see how severe" and then talk to the patient about them after he recovers.

The real life-threatening situation can be completely avoided. The implicit conspiracy of silence commits the staff and patients to isolated positions that sometimes involve the family as well. "Don't talk about upsetting things. Tell him he is looking better." Families are required to deny their concern to alleviate the stress of the patient. All of these maneuvers fend off anxiety, and they allow the staff to stay on neutral topics such as chest pain, palpitations, and fatigue and to ask patients to qualify and quantify these symptoms, while studiously avoiding questions that involve asking the patient what they are thinking about or feeling. The thrust often is to keep the patients cheerful in denial, carefully keeping depression or anxiety out of the coronary care unit.

While denial may at times have adaptive utility in allowing a patient (and staff) to cope, it unfortunately feeds into a psychological set that makes it difficult for the patient to change behavior that directly influences health when he is discharged from the hospital. If one really has not had a serious problem, then why give up smoking, excessive drinking, overeating, type A behavior patterns? Why come to grips with psychological or interpersonal difficulties that may have significantly contributed to the myocardial infarction?

We do not mean to suggest that the entire burden for bringing about these changes rests on the shoulders of the staff, but rather that they have a unique opportunity to begin the process of reorientation that may help a patient change his behavior following discharge from the hospital. Such a change, however, involves a close inspection by the staff of their own personalities, expectations, anxieties, and so forth.

CORONARY CARE UNIT PATIENTS

When one attempts to systematize the psychological structure of the coronary care unit and at the same time enumerate the psychological and interpersonal factors that influence the coronary care unit staff, the equations quickly become highly complex. Coronary care unit patients, it seems, are no less complex. Perhaps by way of introduction we should examine a mythical figure that seems to have been created as coronary care units have evolved, a person who has been frequently labeled "the coronary care unit patient" or "the typical coronary care unit patient." In terms of psychological dynamics, "the coronary care unit patient" simply does not exist.

When patients are unexpectedly plucked out of the mainstream of their lives and suddenly confronted with the imminent possibility of their own death, certain commonalities about such an experience would be shared psychologically by most patients. The same is true for patients' reactions to coronary care units and to the staff of such units. Indeed, the very approach that science dictates in searching for meaning is to seek out common features. The importance of identifying psychological mechanisms is not at issue here. Depression, denial, anxiety, loneliness, hopelessness, and the like are all important psychological feelings that must be identified in coronary patients and their clinical magnitude in coronary care units recognized. Yet at the same time, the search for common patient reactions serves to obscure the incredibly varied group of persons who enter coronary care units. In a scientific sense, this problem can be reduced to a question of statistical variance. How much of the variance of the total possible subjective reactions patients can feel and exhibit in a coronary care unit can be accounted for by the psychological patterns already identified?

This problem of variance can perhaps be clarified by examining analogous situation in which a number of epidemiological studies have been conducted in search of the physiological precursors of coronary disease. These studies have, over the years, been able to identify certain important physiological risk factors such as high blood pressure, obesity, and elevated serum cholesterol that do predicate the subsequent possibility of a myocardial infarction. Yet as valuable as these studies are, the fact remains that these factors account for only a small proportion of the total incidence of coronary disease, clearly suggesting that other unexamined variables still await identification.[10]

In terms of studies on the psychological reactions of coronary care unit patients, no similar, broad-based epidemiological studies have yet been undertaken, so there is no way to accurately gauge how prevalent a response such as depression may be and what it has to do with overall survival within coronary care units. But there is every reason to believe that such studies would be far more complicated than the epidemiological studies on the precursors of coronary disease and the variance accounted for perhaps even less in than those studies.

Patients in coronary care units are similar only to the extent that in one form or another they are all suffering from some form of coronary disease. This does not mean that certain personality types or psychological patterns do not appear more frequently than others, but it does emphasize that the huge variance in coronary patients would serve to mask such a reality even if it were a very potent variable. Elderly patients suffering from a degenerative process can be seen in almost any coronary care unit next to a 35-year-old male, who would be judged by the casual observer to be in remarkably "good shape." In many urban hospitals, a lawyer, judge, or physician can be seen resting in a bed next to an indigent. Such variance mitigates against overall or generalized prescriptive psychological advice and suggests that, in spite of its pitfalls, there is a critical need on the part of the staff for common sense sprinkled liberally with large doses of human compassion.

Having emphasized that no individual patient can be construed to be an epidemiological statistic or a conglomeration of psychological constructs, we will discuss one psychosocial factor that leads certain types of persons to be over-represented in coronary care units—interpersonal factors that lead to human loneliness and premature coronary disease. The destructive impact of human loneliness and its relationship to premature death has been described by Lynch.[15] Between the critical ages of 35 and 64 years, those who live alone, whether male or female, white or nonwhite, have statistically significant higher death rates than those who are married (Table 5). A large number of clinical case studies, as well as population statistics, all point toward the conclusion that human loneliness contributes to the development of coronary disease.[15] In similar fashion, those interpersonal difficulties within marriages that frequently lead to divorce also seem to contribute to coronary disease.[15] As a result, many patients in coronary care units are in fact either lonely or experiencing interpersonal problems long before they come to a hospital.

A nurse or physician who enters a patient's life in the coronary care unit does so midstream and in a very transient fashion. Yet the entrance is also unavoidably

Table 5. Death rates for coronary heart disease per 100,000 population by age, color, sex, and marital status, U.S. 1959-1961

	35-44	45-54	55-64
White males			
Married	81	330	849
Single	119	458	1088
Widowed	149	548	1314
Divorced	200	713	1634
White females			
Married	12	60	254
Single	25	80	263
Widowed	28	102	376
Divorced	25	96	331
Nonwhite males			
Married	78	257	643
Single	159	456	858
Widowed	203	683	1443
Divorced	188	596	1226
Nonwhite females			
Married	41	148	371
Single	76	205	426
Widowed	100	318	772
Divorced	56	208	518

From Lynch, J. J.: The broken heart: the medical consequences of loneliness, New York, 1977, Basic Books, Inc., Publishers.

interpersonal and, as Klein et al.[13] suggest, quite meaningful for patients. As has been documented elsewhere,[16,19,21,23] even interactions as transient and as apparently routine as a nurse palpating a patient's pulse seem to take on special significance. The effects of such brief interactions can be objectively measured in patient heart reactions. For example, in examining the cardiac responses of over 200 coronary patients to repeated pulse palpation, we found that even this routine interaction significantly reduced the incidence of ventricular arrhythmia in those patients exhibiting high frequencies of such ectopic beats.[18] To show that such reactions are not secondary to changes in respiration or physical movement, we monitored heart reactions of comatose patients in a hospital shock-trauma unit[17] who were totally paralyzed by d-tubocurarine and supported by respirators. Even these patients showed heart rate changes of up to 30 beats per minute when a nurse held their hand and comforted them. Without delving further into the psychophysiology of such reactions here, these data demonstrate that even the most routine aspects of clinical care and bedside manner have measurable effects on the hearts of coronary patients.

In summary, the coronary care unit, its staff, and its patients are viewed by us as one cross section of our modern scientific culture. The environment is one that brings to bear all of the best available technology and clinical competence to aggressively treat the damaged heart. Most clinical staffs seem to be intuitively aware of the larger sociopsychological milieu of the coronary patients in their units, but the very structure of compartmentalized care makes it difficult for staffs to believe they can do anything clinically effective about these larger problems. Part of the solution to this problem must involve changing the health consciousness of our entire society; in a certain sense it involves a revolution in the way we think about coronary disease and health. People in general must understand that cardiac health, especially in the context of coronary care units, involves similar commitment of care beyond the coronary care unit. To that extent, cardiovascular health involves many medical issues that go far beyond scientific determinism.

Even in such an environment as a coronary care unit, once the link between the world of the unit and the larger patient "world" is seen, it does become easier to revise one's clinical approach to patients. If part of the solution involves altering the consciousness of our society, then most certainly the consciousness of individual patients can be altered by the coronary care unit staff. If we have fragmented such problems at a cultural level—disconnected heart disease in the coronary care unit from such pandemic problems as human loneliness—then we have done the very same thing to individual patients.

REFERENCES

1. Broughton, R., and Baron, R.: Sleep of acute coronary patients in an open ward intensive care unit, Sleep Res. **2:**144, 1973.
2. Cassem, N.: The nurse in the coronary care unit: psychological aspects of myocardial infarction and coronary care, St. Louis, 1975, The C. V. Mosby Co.
3. Deamer, R. M., Scharf, M., and Kales, A.: Sleep patterns in the coronary care unit, U.S. Navy Med. **59:**19, 1972.
4. Dohno, S., et al.: Some aspects of sleep disturbances in coronary care patients, Percept. Mot. Skills **48:**199, 1979.
5. Gentry, W. D., Foster, S. B., and Froehling, S.: Psychological response to situational stress in intensive and non-intensive nursing, Heart Lung **1:**793, 1972.
6. Gross, H. S.: The effects of race and sex on the variation of diagnosis and disposition in a psychiatric emergency room, J. Nerv. Ment. Dis. **148:**638, 1969.
7. Gross, H. S.: A psychodynamic meaning of doctor-patient relationships, Psychodynamic Foundations of Medicine, **2:**199, 1978.
8. Hackett, T. P., and Cassem, N. H.: The psychology of intensive care: problems and their management, New York, 1977, Brunner/Mazel, Inc.
9. Hackett, T. P., Cassem, N. H., and Wishnie, H. A.: The coronary care unit: an appraisal of its psychological hazards, N. Engl. J. Med. **279:**1365, 1968.
10. Jenkins, C. D.: Psychologic and social precursors of coronary disease (first of two parts), N. Engl. J. Med. **282:**244, 1971.
11. Jewitt, D. E., et al.: Free noradrenaline and adrenaline excretion in relation to the development of cardiac arrhythmias and heart failure patients with acute myocardial infarction, Lancet **i:**636, 1969.
12. Karacan, I., et al.: Sleep in post myocardial infarction patients, contemporary problems in cardiology: stress and the heart, Mt. Kisco, N.Y., 1974, Futura Publications.
13. Klein, R. F., et al.: Transfer from a coronary care unit, Arch. Intern. Med. **122:**104, 1968.
14. Lesher, S.: After a heart attack: there comes a will to live—well, New York Times Magazine, p. 9, January 27, 1974.
15. Lynch, J. J.: The broken heart: the medical consequences of loneliness, New York, 1977, Basic Books, Inc., Publishers.

16. Lynch, J. J., et al.: The effects of human contact on cardiac arrhythmia in coronary care patients, J. Nerv. Ment. Dis. **158:**88, 1974.
17. Lynch, J. J., et al.: Effects of human contact on the heart activity of curarized patients in a shock-trauma unit, Am. Heart J. **88:**160, 1974.
18. Lynch, J. J., et al.: Human contact and cardiac arrhythmia in coronary care unit, Psychosom. Med. **39:**188, 1977.
19. Lynch, J. J., et al.: Psychological aspects of cardiac arrhythmias, Am. Heart J. **93:**645, 1977.
20. Miller, W. B., and Rosenfeld, R.: A psychophysiological study of denial following acute myocardial infarction, J. Psychosom. Res. **19:**43, 1975.
21. Mills, M. A., et al.: Effect of pulse palpation on cardiac arrhythmia in coronary care patients, Nurs. Res. **25:**378, 1976.
22. Orne, M. T.: On the social psychology of the psychological experiment: with particular reference to demand characteristics and their implications, Am. Psychol. **17:**776, 1962.
23. Thomas, S. A., Lynch, J. J., and Mills, M. E.: Psychosocial influences on heart arrhythmia in coronary care patients, Heart Lung **4:**746, 1975.
24. Valori, C., Thomas, M., and Shillingford, J.: Free noradrenaline and adrenaline excretion in relation to clinical syndromes following myocardial infarction, Am. J. Cardiol. **20:**605, 1967.

6

The nurse in the coronary care unit

NED H. CASSEM
KRISTINE NELSON
R. R. RICH

Ventricular fibrillation is always a disconcerting event in the coronary care unit, but when it occurred in a patient who was a Nobel laureate, it was shocking. Stable up to that day, his third in the unit, and asking permission to give his annual lecture to the medical students 2 days later, the professor, without warning, developed a run of rapid ventricular tachycardia that swiftly deteriorated into ventricular fibrillation. No physicians were in the unit at the time, and a code call was sounded as two nurses brought the defibrillator to his bedside. When the first physician appeared moments later, the patient's normal sinus rhythm had been restored. The news of the professor's arrest spread quickly, and faces in the unit mirrored shock, dismay, disbelief, and relief at his close call with death. As the excitement faded, attention returned to the continuous EKG tracing that told the story of the event. The total time elapsed between onset of ventricular tachycardia and the restoration of normal sinus rhythm had been 11 seconds.

Dramatic for the coronary care unit nurses? Yes, but routine. Patients' tension, recurrent pain, life-threatening arrhythmias, extended infarcts, family conflicts, the breathlessness of acute pulmonary edema, monitor alarms, potent and dangerous intravenous infusions, therapeutic triumphs, and lingering deaths are all a part of the daily happenings in a coronary care unit. While ventricular fibrillation is countershocked, alarms attended to, arrhythmias recorded and treated, and infusions closely monitored, the nurses also take responsibility for reducing the emotional distress of the patients and for helping them better understand coronary disease and its management. Simultaneously, they cooperate to bolster and maintain their own morale as they meet these multiple professional responsibilities.

TAKING CARE OF THE PATIENT

In a study of the reactions of patients to coronary care unit nurses, patients were asked to list the qualities they considered most important in the nurses who took care of them.[3] The most frequently mentioned characteristics were cheerfulness, competence, understanding, efficiency, kindness, and tenderness. Patients placed most emphasis, however, on the immediate attention and close watch provided by the nurses. Pentecost et al.[9] have also stated that the constant presence of the nurses was the outstanding source of reassurance to patients in the coronary care unit. As one patient said, "I wish our fire department would answer calls the way they do!" In fact, patients involved in this study commonly compared nurses' responses to their alarms and call buttons to the response of fire departments to fire alarms. The nurses made good use of this and repeatedly reminded the patients that someone was always on hand and that their condition was constantly being monitored.

Competence encourages a feeling of security in patients and can alone be a source of reassurance. When asked about the nursing care he had received, one patient singled out a nurse who had been in a rather bad mood during his time in the coronary care unit. "Oh, she's a tough one, she is! Her husband must have to watch his step! But is it good to have her near by—she really knows what she's doing!" There is no substitute for competence. As Ferrigan has said, "The entire success of intensive coronary care is dependent on the competence of the nurse."[6]

One of the more harrowing experiences for the nurse just beginning her coronary care unit experience is having to learn at the bedside. Not only are nurses aware of their uncertainties about monitoring equipment and procedures, but they also can feel keenly the occasional insecurities that this produces in patients. It is not at all helpful when some of the more frightened patients actually express their doubts. At times this felt mistrust can be a projection on the part of the nurse, because the patient is more likely to take a cue from the mood of the nurse than from the actual fact of orientation or the presence of a "teacher."

The two most common emotional problems with which coronary care patients and their nurses must cope are fear and depression. A patient may fear that he is on the verge of dying, or he may feel that "something bad" is about to happen, for example, recurrent pain, breathlessness, or a vague, unspecified event that is worse that anything he has already experienced.

Fear in coronary patients is best treated initially by emphasizing the positive features of the coronary care unit. The constant vigilance of the staff and the role of the monitoring equipment may be explained as safeguards of the patient's welfare.

Few staff members forget to introduce themselves by name to a patient at the first meeting. Because the memories of most coronary patients can be impaired by physical discomfort, anxiety, and age, it remains important to reintroduce oneself by name on two or three subsequent meetings.

The sooner the family is introduced to coronary care procedures, the better. As soon as the patient has been settled in the unit, the family can be brought into the room and, in their presence, the patient can be instructed about the monitoring equipment. (If he has already been told or it is his second admission, family instruction provides an excellent occasion for the patient to hear again these important facts.) Movement artifacts on the monitor and false alarms can be explained and deliberately demonstrated to prepare patient and family for their occurrence. All should know that regular measurement of vital signs and an indwelling intravenous line are routine in the coronary care unit. Patients should be specifically told how often their vital signs will be taken and that the intravenous line is present for delivery of any medication the patient may need. The combined message of the monitor and intravenous line is that the coronary care unit personnel are constantly prepared to take care of the patient's needs.

The patient's own contribution to monitoring is then explained. His role is to report immediately to the nurse any chest pain, no matter how trivial it seems to him. He is told he will be asked to judge the severity of his pain from 0 (no pain at all) to 10 (the worst pain I've ever had). Then an EKG will be taken before medication for the pain, which is right at hand, can be given. When the pain is gone, another EKG will be taken. In this way, it can be determined whether the pain comes from the heart and whether treatment helps it. The patient and his family who have received this type of orientation to the coronary care unit environment and routine should be able to derive a feeling of security rather than apprehension from the presence and functioning of the staff and the equipment. Once this point is reached, the nursing staff can begin to help the patient be aware of and able to deal with the fears related to his illness.

In general the therapeutic rule for treating fear is to base any approach on indications from the patient rather than to probe blindly for hidden anxieties. For example, if a patient is reluctant to fall asleep it is reasonable to assume that his hesitation may stem from a fear that sleep will somehow make him more vulnerable to death. The nurse might ask the patient whether he is having trouble falling asleep. The patient may say yes but does not know why. It is neither helpful nor necessary to tell a patient he may be afraid of death, but one could ask if any of his recent symptoms came during the night. Even if he denies this, it is all right to say, "It is natural for anyone to have trouble sleeping in a new or strange place. That is why doctors here always order a mild sleeping pill. Some people think they are not supposed to sleep because problems can be recognized only if they are awake and can tell us about them. All our monitors work just as well when you're asleep as when you are wide awake. In fact, if you can relax and sleep, it will help your heart because it is more restful." (This is untrue only for those patients who experience angina during some REM sleep periods.)

Medication is often a valuable adjunct in dealing with patients' fears and anxieties. Medication orders should be written for a dosage range to be administered at regular intervals, for example, 2 to 5 mg of diazepam every 4 hours. Since nurses who are constantly in touch with the patient are the best judges of his level of anxiety, the most effective regulation of sedation can be achieved through their evaluation of the patient's needs.

Unlike fear, depression usually develops when a patient's condition has stabilized and he has begun to think about the implications of a myocardial infarction. A damaged heart is a severe blow to self-esteem, so that a myocardial infarction is often followed by an "ego infarction." The typical ruminations are familiar to coronary care unit nurses. "I'm washed up. I won't be able to take care of my family, my job is in danger, I'm just not the same—getting old and falling apart. I won't be able to drive, exercise, play sports, I won't be able to satisfy my wife sexually, I'll have to stop smoking and give up what I like to eat. I've had it. What a rotten life!" Typical was an accountant, 40 years of age, who cheerily said that his admission had been a "big hoax." He had been healthy all his life, he said, so that his friends even referred to him as "the bull," but as he talked he grew serious and his face fell. "When I get back home, I'll be walking down the street and someone will point me out and whisper, 'There goes another guy with a heart attack at the age of 40—check him off the list!'"

The ability to listen and draw out specific concerns in this area is the mark of an especially skillful nurse. Charted notes of the patient's verbalized concerns (in his exact words) can be of great value in the staff's effort to relate to the patient as a whole person. For example, a note that says, "The patient appeared anxious and discussed dying with me; after this he seemed calmer . . ." is not only vague but may evoke criticism from a physician who has not been told accurately enough how such a "discussion" arose. A more accurate note would say: "After the lidocaine drip was increased to 2 mg/min, the patient asked, 'Am I going to make it?' He was reassured that his condition remained under control. He then said his brother, after his myocardial infarction, had died suddenly in an intensive care unit when everything looked stable. I explained to him that each heart attack is unique and that his should not be equated with his brother's. He seemed calmer after this." Few physicians can quarrel with what patients utter spontaneously. The best convalescent plans are built when specific vulnerabilities are kept in mind. It is very important to know why a patient believes that certain evils will befall him. Even so, involvement in these types of patient problems requires a costly investment in both time and emotion. Psychological intervention is discussed in greater detail in Chapter 10.

Patient teaching in the coronary care unit

Although information given to patients during the acute phase is not fully retained, the actual time spent sitting down with patients and their families communicates a genuine sense of caring on the part of the nurse. Listening carefully, the nurse must be tuned in to cues that indicate a request for information. A statement from the patient during the early course following a myocardial infarction such as "I guess this means I won't be returning to work" is one that the nurse should explore with the patient.

The major goal of patient teaching must always be kept in mind. Teaching serves as a catalyst of adaptation to illness, during which the patient grows and changes. It examines existing alternatives, relieves doubts, and clarifies misconceptions.[13] "Learning" for the patient means changing his behavior, knowledge, values, and attitudes. Simply supplying a neatly packaged program comprised of guidelines, protocols, and teaching tools will not produce change. The patient must be "ready, willing, and able" to change.[4] These prerequisites are not always encountered in the coronary care unit, but the nurse should evaluate the patient with these in mind. Although the patient may not be in a state of "readiness," the nurse is still able at this time to assess factors such as intellectual level, health beliefs, and availability of support systems that will ultimately affect the teaching plan. The following objectives and outcomes, based on the A.N.A. Standards of Cardiovascular Nursing Practice, can serve as guidelines in assessing patients and planning for discharge. It must be emphasized that because each coronary patient is a unique individual, their outcomes must be specifically tailored to their expectations. By the time of discharge the patient will:

I. Demonstrate a knowledge level that will enable him to make appropriate therapeutic judgments and seek medical help when indicated
   A. Accurately describe what to do if chest pain occurs
   B. Describe the signs and symptoms that necessitate medical advice such as
      1. Chest pain unrelieved by nitroglycerin and rest
      2. Increased shortness of breath
      3. Fainting
      4. Very slow or rapid heart rate
   C. Be able to accurately take own pulse
   D. State time, date, place, and person(s) to be seen for follow-up care
II. Maintain a pharmacological regimen that is compatible with therapeutic and personal goals
   A. State when to take each medication
   B. Describe desired effects of each medication
   C. Describe possible adverse reactions to each medication
   D. Describe what to do if adverse reactions to medication occur
III. Maintain a dietary intake that is compatible with therapeutic and personal goals
   A. Describe dietary restrictions
   B. Describe rationale for restrictions

C. State examples of foods to avoid
D. State that excessive body weight increases the work of the heart
E. Describe the effects of alcohol on the heart
F. Describe the effects of coffee on the heart

IV. Demonstrate a knowledge level that will enable him to appropriately modify his life style
A. Describe an infarction and describe angina
B. Identify risk factors and relate them to the development of coronary disease
C. Identify own risk factors
D. Indicate an understanding of the importance of providing the heart with adequate oxygen and rest by describing factors that decrease oxygen supply and/or increase work load
1. Digestion of food
2. Cigarette smoking
3. Emotional stress
4. Very hot or cold weather
5. Very hot or cold baths or showers
6. Isometric exercises (gives examples of these)
7. Working with arms above shoulder level

V. Participate in the planning of modification of life-style
A. Describe own plan for the resumption of the following activities that is consistent with prescribed activity level
1. Activities of daily living
2. Household tasks
3. Sexual activity
4. Vocational activities
5. Driving a car
6. Recreation
B. Discuss plan to decrease or stop cigarette smoking
C. Discuss plan to minimize or eliminate sources of stress and tension
D. Discuss and implement plan to screen children for risk factors

VI. Demonstrate effective coping mechanisms to adapt to his altered life-style
A. Able to cope with anxiety as evidenced by the following
1. Sleep at least 6 hours in a 24-hour period without interruption
2. Body musculature is relaxed during rest periods
3. Talk about events other than those related to self or own illness
4. Resume grooming behavior

VII. Maintain activity pattern that is compatible with therapeutic and personal goals
   A. Describe factors that should be taken into account when walking
      1. Distance
      2. Speed
      3. Weather
      4. Incline
   B. Discuss plan for walking and outline stages of progression

If the patient, while still in the coronary care unit, has indicated that he indeed wants to change to "prevent this thing from happening again," his motivation may be enhanced by contracting with the nurse for the learning or behavior change. A contract states what the patient must do to achieve the objective ("will not resume cigarette smoking') and what the nurse will do ("will visit the patient daily until discharge and make one follow-up telephone call a month for 3 months"). The concept of behavior change contracts is based on principles of adult education and change theory.[4]

Patient teaching, formal and informal, occupies a great deal of the coronary care unit nurse's time. And rightfully so. The opportunities for patient teaching in this area are plentiful. As noted above, careful and sensitive explanations given by the nurse at the time of admission to the unit can serve to reduce fear.[3] Incidental, explanatory teaching during the patient's stay will increase his sense of well-being. Teaching deep breathing exercises and use of the footboard during routine care and identifying medications by name when administering them are but a few examples.

Educational preparation of the patient for procedures and events such as cardiac catheterization and transfer from the unit is an expectation of the coronary care unit nurse. Family members should be included. They can be recipients of the nurse's teaching in a variety of ways: instructions enabling them to assist with the patient's care when appropriate, explanations of the rationale for visitors' restrictions, and reassuring progress reports by the patient's own nurse.

Patient teaching is a responsibility of the nursing staff. More recent evidence indicates that patient teaching by nurses can increase the patient's knowledge and return to work and improve adherence to discharge instructions.[10] Teaching, even about threatening subjects, can decrease anxiety. While training families of coronary patients in cardiopulmonary resuscitation and monitoring reports of the spouse about feelings of power and control, Nelson demonstrated a decrease in anxiety levels.[8] Many further investigations of nursing intervention through teaching remain to be done so that this powerful force for patient benefit can be maximized.

Table 6. Combined frequency and severity of conflicts experienced by coronary care unit nurses

Combined score	Item
57	Heavy lifting
46	Intra-aortic balloon pump research
44	Unpredictable scheduling; weight of personal responsibility
42	Family overwrought and anxious
40	Hectic pace
38	Family annoys staff
36	Patient's illness is severe or prognosis is poor; not enough time off; poor time scheduling
35	Personal feeling of insecurity
34	Troublesome patient behavior or personality
31	Personality conflicts with other nurses
30	Elderly patients are depressing; unavailability of physicians; poor communication with physicians

TAKING CARE OF THE STAFF

There are inevitably situations in which it is necessary for nurses to inflict pain on patients, for example, when the patient must cough or turn, receive an injection, or undergo suctioning. In such circumstances, which are routine in the coronary care unit, it is often difficult to maintain a balance between empathic concern for the patient and the personal toughness and resilience necessary for continued effectiveness. This is typical of the type of demand made of coronary care unit nurses, and it is only one of the job requirements that creates stress and necessitates attention to the needs of staff as well as patients in the coronary care unit.

Cassem and Hackett[2] conducted a study in which they met weekly for discussions with a group of coronary care unit nurses. A list of 44 problems mentioned during these meetings was kept, and the nurses subsequently were given this list and asked to rank the items according to the frequency of occurrence and severity of stress that each produced. Table 6 lists the items ranked as being most stressful and occurring most often. The 16 nurses who participated were surprised to find that heavy lifting was ranked most often as a major source of stress.* This is an interesting result in view of the tendency to emphasize primarily emotional issues. It should also be pointed out that this study was done at a time when the intra-aortic balloon pump was first introduced in the coronary care unit. It was used at that time only for patients in end-stage cardiogenic shock, and

*Although only one nurse had undergone lumbar laminectomy and fusion in the 6 years since the inception of the coronary care unit, the number of backaches per staff member has never been calculated.

only one of the first ten patients so treated survived. This undoubtedly influenced the high level of negative response to this procedure. Since that time the intra-aortic balloon pump has become a welcome intervention for cardiogenic shock and unstable angina. Years of medical research have proved its efficacy. In our experience, we have seen a confidence develop in caring for patients with the intra-aortic balloon pump. One factor that may be responsible for this development is directly related to the increased hospital survival of patients having been treated with this counterpulsation device. Ten years of experience with balloon pumping has led to a more refined screening process for the selection of patients. The efforts of these earlier nurses and their successors laid the foundation for the development of educational programs describing the physiologic and psychologic aspects of care of these patients. Technological advancements have also increased the challenge in caring for these patients.

As listed in the study by Cassem and Hackett,[2] anxiety of patient's families was regarded by the nurses as a major source of stress. We maintain that nurses presently working in coronary care units experience this as a frequent source of conflict. The nurse faces the dilemma of meeting the constant physical demands of the critically ill patient while at the same time effectively providing emotional support for the family.

In a second part of this study seven general areas of concern were selected; these were families, patients, physicians, other nurses, research procedures, nursing administration, and scheduling and staffing. The nurses were asked to compare these items two at a time, selecting the one responsible for producing greater stress. Results of these comparisons are presented in Table 7. The fact that the nursing administration and scheduling problems are listed as primary sources of stress suggests that factors such as scapegoating might have played a role in the rating.

Starting in 1972 one of us (NHC) began to meet weekly with the nurses of this same coronary care unit staff for the purpose of exploring in greater depth the sources of stress to which staff members were subject. In addition to these weekly meetings I made it a point to be present at the daily 2:30 P.M. report whenever a cardiac arrest, death, or an unusual source of stress had occurred. The staff was asked to share reactions to such an event at that time. The issues raised can be divided into two general problem areas, sources of stress related to patients and sources of stress related to staff.

Patients as sources of conflict

Although behavior problems can be quite troublesome from time to time, coronary patients are most threatening to us as coronary care unit staff when they are very sick, very old, or very young. Probably the most intense stress is generated by dying patients. Price and Bergen suggest that coronary care unit nurses

Table 7. General areas of conflict in the coronary care unit*

Rank	Source	Score
1	Nursing administration	67.0
2	Scheduling and staffing	61.2
3	Families	36.5
4	Research procedures	33.5
5	Other nurses	31.5
6	Patients	25.0
7	Physicians	17.0

*From Cassem, N. H., and Hackett, T. P.: Am. J. Nurs. **17**:1426, 1972.

may suffer from "the unconscious blurring of the boundary between an awareness of being responsible for the care of an ill or dying patient and the feeling of being responsible for the occurrence of the patient's illness or death."[11] This is not viewed as psychiatric pathology or a "hang-up" but rather as stress that is peculiar to the times. As medical and technological interventions increase, so can the moral-ethical issues that are inherent in the care of the sick. Simon and Whitely have reported how feelings of hopelessness and confusion about how to respond to the dying patient and the patient's family can be responsible for the anxiety and tension that develop when caring for terminally ill persons.[12]

Technological advances have also brought opportunities for nurses to learn how to care for terminally ill patients. The willingness to assist the irreversibly ill patient has markedly increased. A 35-year-old father of two children suffered a massive anterior myocardial infarction and required the intra-aortic balloon pump for stabilization. Angiograms showed inoperable triple-vessel coronary disease. His ventricular function was dependent on the balloon pump. Although fully alert, the man remained sullen and withdrawn and communicated very little with anyone, but did somewhat more with his wife. In group meetings, the nurses' observations were shared, and because the patient seemed much calmer in his wife's presence, the nurses decided to focus maximum support on her (who did respond warmly to them) so that she might have greater support to maintain vigil until her husband's death. Despite the difficult feeling left by the patient's condition, the nurses maintained a constant support for his wife so that she was able to remain with him for the 3 days prior to his death. The nurses remained with her after his death as well. It was support she never forgot.

Use of group meetings

Four ingredients are required for an effective group session.

1. The feeling of at least one individual about a patient or patient care issue must be identified (for example, anxiety, guilt, or anger).
2. The group members must react to the feeling with their own response. In

addition to one person's being open enough to identify a feeling state toward a patient or an event, other group members must make the effort to be equally open and honest about their own reactions (for example, those who admitted they also feared rupturing the patient's aneurysm).

3. Some critical perspective must be achieved through the group process. The event or feeling about a patient must be critically reviewed, with appropriate support, praise, and planning added.
4. Appropriate resolution or integration must follow. At times it is sufficient to identify successes and failures associated with a traumatic event such as an arrest. Usually these are learning experiences from which the nurse emerges with either practical suggestions or a more complete perspective on a problem. The nurse who had been slow to respond to the arrest did not have the problem again. She realized she did not have to worry about the respect of her fellow nurses but only about her personal vulnerability in forming attachments.

Meetings can also be used to assist staff members in coping with behavioral problems presented by patients. A 40-year-old patient who looked more like a Marlboro man than a person with end-stage left ventricular function returned to the coronary care unit 9 months after his initial admission for a massive anterior myocardial infarction. Kept in the coronary care unit for 3 full weeks the first time, he had been very well liked by the whole staff, had occasionally dropped in on his return visits to the hospital, and had never been any problem. This time, however, Karen, a nurse who had liked him before, was furious with him. His statements had become quite sexually explicit, but she was angered most by his calling her "Legs." When this was presented to the other nurses, two verified that his statements had been much more forward. At that point he had not touched anyone, but references to sex abounded in his conversation. Some nurses had not noticed this in his speech; one laughed and said she felt excluded. We all recalled how devoted he was to his wife. The key to the mystery was supplied in the history taken by the house officer, in which he had mentioned that in the month prior to the current admission the patient's efforts at intercourse had been accompanied by angina and shortness of breath. The patient was extremely worried that someone would tell his wife this and repeatedly emphasized to the house officer his desire not to have it made known. His behavior therefore represented not primary eroticism but sexualized fear. Simply discovering him to be a threatened man changed Karen's perspective and some of her feelings toward him, but several suggestions were also made for confronting his behavior. (She had been so angry she had said nothing to him up to this point.) Suggestions included asking him whether he realized that his speech contained so many references to sex and simply telling him that she preferred to be called by her own name rather than "Legs." When she mentioned this to the patient later, he actually began to discuss his worries over his inability to care for his wife. He was no problem for Karen after that.

How staff create their own stress

Of all the sources of conflict among staff members, probably the most serious stems from excessive competition. There is a normal, healthy need in all of us to be recognized as competent and worthwhile. Coronary care unit personnel are often (and usually like to be) recognized as supercompetent. When properly channeled, this motivation is a powerful stimulus to superior performance. However, as self-esteem falters, more primitive instincts struggle for the upper hand. When most of us are feeling inferior, we may succumb to the temptation to boost our egos by putting somebody else down.

Self-esteem can be easily damaged. The coronary care unit nurse may not want temporary assignment to the general wards, and when this is a necessity such a nurse may feel insufficiently recognized as a capable person on the new unit or that she was singled out from other staff to "float" for unknown reasons. A "float list" may help to ease some of these feelings. All the staffs' names are included on the list, and people are chosen to float to other units based on the last date an individual floated. This way, floating is shared equally among the staff; no one is singled out.

Personnel from other units may respond antagonistically, describing coronary care unit nurses as prima donnas who are overrated and underworked. ("Their staff-patient ratio is practically one to one and here we are, three nurses for 40 patients.") Friday afternoon transfers from the coronary care unit to other parts of the hospital are often labeled "dumps" by those on the receiving end. This could be aggravated if patients leaving the coronary care unit are poorly prepared for the reduced attention they receive from the nursing staff on other floors. Nurses to whom they are sent often hear how poorly their services compare with those offered in the coronary care unit. The coronary care unit nurse may be criticized as arrogant by other nurses before they know anything about her personally. The more insecure the nurse who transfers the patient from the coronary care unit, the more likely she is to regard the receiving nurse as incapable of carrying out or perhaps even understanding the transfer orders. Some of these situations, even though they sound almost childish, are quite common; the remedy is better communication. We do not often enough refer to the underlying cause, namely that someone thinks he or she has to appear better. We have a perverse tendency to try to make ourselves feel better by regarding others as somehow inferior. The second major principle is that the less self-esteem people have, the more they are likely to insist on being regarded as somehow superior. The corollary: the most secure and competent people generate the least friction.

Coronary care unit nurses are not immune to stereotyping behavior. Nurses who are temporarily assigned to the unit may suddenly become aware that their unfamiliarity with the unit is being italicized by the not very subtle maneuvers of a coronary care unit nurse. ("Suddenly I'm being watched as though I were a menace in here," one complained.) As a group, those hardest on the floats tend to be the less experienced coronary care unit nurses. Once the occasion arose for a group of coronary care unit nurses to become highly specialized and form a research team to study cardiogenic shock. Even though they had been coronary care unit nurses themselves, these nurses were now criticized as prima donnas who led a privileged life, thought they knew it all, and frequently "dumped" patients in the coronary care unit on Friday nights merely because they had social engagements to attend. Similar types of alienation can arise between shifts of the same staff, especially the night shift, whose members often tend to be permanent and are therefore set apart with fewer avenues of communication available with the remainder of the staff.

Excessive competition does the greatest damage at the personal level within the unit itself. Once when I walked into the unit one of the nurses whispered, "I don't know what's going on in here today. Everybody wants to be in charge." In the struggle for rank in the pecking order, the newest nurse is most likely to be put down. Surprisingly insulting comments may be heard when a (or especially more than one) new staff person arrives ("I've got the weekend to look forward to, and I'm all alone with Mary and a float!"). Feeling already insecure, the newest nurse is thus often made to feel more a liability than an asset in the coronary care unit, and there is a tendency for that nurse to pass the stigma and the problem along to the next new nurse who joins the unit staff. Although the new nurse is the person most in need of support and help, a person in this position may (if times are very bad) become a convenient scapegoat for everyone else's feelings of inadequacy.

An astute head nurse can help to ward off some of the stigmata associated with being a new staff person. Recognizing the new staff member's prior experience as an asset in adapting to the new environment builds confidence. Delegating the responsibility of some of the newer staff member's orientation to a senior staff nurse lessens the threat of transition while recognizing the senior nurse for her expertise. This tends to decrease any tendency to scapegoat a new person because the senior nurse now has an investment in the new nurse's experience and strives to make the adaptation period pleasant. This tends to have a "snowball" effect as more nurses share in the orientation of newer staff members. It is the responsibility of the head nurse, however, to ensure that a standard orientation program is followed. This will decrease the risk of confusion for the new staff nurse caused by multiple persons involved in the orientation process.

A hazing period for the newest members is normal in most closely organized groups. When "hazing" becomes generalized or malignant, however, the sources must be sought elsewhere. Usually they are found in the relationship of the head nurse or the supervisor to the staff. The most common setting is one in which criticism has almost entirely replaced praise as the major means of unit reinforcement. Guilt is high, tempers are short, and everyone is "mistake-conscious." The more insecure the head nurse makes her staff feel, the more the newest nurse is likely to suffer.

How conflicts are masked

Scapegoating is a way of life. Just as frustrations can be taken out on individuals, so too inordinate amounts of heat and energy can be expended on issues that may themselves be trivial. Efficiency and cleanliness are convenient banners to wave when the participants are angry or upset about something else. One can recognize that the real problem may lie elsewhere when notes on the scut sheet start to take on a nasty tone ("Whoever had 412 and 413 last night left them a shambles"). We only leave notes like this when our anger is deeper and more generalized. When individuals or entire shifts begin to feel that they are the only ones who "care" about the unit or about the patients, trouble is brewing. The issue is not neatness in the unit but rather intrastaff alienation.

What about patients who "are not allowed to die with dignity"? A very legitimate problem in itself, this issue can become a lightning rod on which other problems and frustrations are discharged. The most common issue hidden by this complaint is the unavoidable death of a particularly well-liked or young patient. The day after the death of a 35-year-old man with a myocardial infarction and inoperable coronary artery disease, the nurses presented a request to talk about Mrs. R. Mrs. R. was a patient who had been transferred from another intensive care unit to our coronary care unit to have a Swann-Ganz catheter put in place. It was not at all for her benefit, the nurses argued, but just another procedure performed to satisfy the physicians' curiosity. Not only did it cause her more distress, but it robbed her of a possibly more peaceful death. As legitimate as it was to discuss that issue, it was important to know why the topic arose at that moment, since Mrs. R. had been in the unit 8 months earlier. As the nurses began to talk about it, the conversation returned to the efforts to resuscitate the young man the day before. Overdrive pacing had been our last resort in attempting to control his ventricular tachycardia. The effort had failed and had seemed to make him suffer more. Yet no one could think of how we could have avoided any of the treatment measures carried out the day before. The bitter frustration of failure still smarted. In these circumstances it was very natural to raise the issue of Mrs. R. When there is no legitimate object for all our feelings of frustration and anger, we search for the most convenient object on which to vent our feelings. For that reason, whenever angry cries are raised about prolonging life in unsalvageable patients (especially if the incidence of such cases has not changed), it is worthwhile to find out if a young person has died recently despite a resuscitation effort.

Scapegoating upward is a favorite sport, as all who hold higher office know. That the nursing administration and problems with scheduling could rank so far ahead of other possible sources of conflict (Table 7) suggests that other issues remained hidden. Most of them focus on fear (often mutual fear) or the feeling of being devalued by one's superiors. It is important for head nurses, supervisors, and directors to remember that they "cannot win." Once the staff suggested to a head nurse that she take a more active hand in patient care activities in the coronary care unit. One nurse suggested that when the head nurse came into the room and saw items in disarray or dirty laundry, she might help by straightening up, provided she had time. In the next group meeting it was learned that the head nurse had tried this, but as she had taken a basin of dirty water from a patient's room to empty it the staff nurse appeared to be insulted and said, "*I* can do it!" as though the head nurse's gesture were a criticism of her inefficiency or incompetence. This outcome seems to indicate that in this case the staff may well have been seeking something other than active assistance from the head nurse. Behind such conflicts is a desire on the part of the staff for the head nurse to care about them and respect their abilities. There is also a feeling that the head nurse should not be too aloof or detached from direct patient care. The head nurse who pitches in from time to time "like a regular" appears to minimize these fears more effectively. Once the staff becomes accustomed to the head nurse's continued assistance with patient care, such comments begin to decline.

Of course the head nurse and supervisor are still expected to be supercompetent. The belief that someone nearby knows what to do in case of a disaster generates more security than most people usually care to admit. It may be no accident that with head nurses off duty, evening supervisors seem to be criticized more often for lack of familiarity with the equipment, procedures, or complicated emergencies arising in the coronary care unit. The competent coronary care unit nurse does not want constant guidance in routine care delivery, but appreciates the security of being able to consult with someone with greater expertise whenever in doubt. It can also be hard for a supervisor to overcome a stereotype of incompetence. One of our best coronary care unit nurses became a supervisor on the evening shift. When a cardiac arrest occurred, she was the first nurse to reach the scene but found that the house officer communicated with her only reluctantly as they proceeded with the early stages of resuscitation. With the arrival of the nurse from the coronary care unit who was assigned to code calls, the house officer showed immediate and great relief and began to ask this nurse all the same questions he had asked the supervisor, whom he now totally ignored.

Fear and suspicion between administration and staff at times reaches the level of mild paranoia. The administration in such circumstances is usually described as flinging down unilateral decisions without any interest in the opinions of or consultation with those who will have to live with the changes and make them work. On the other hand, should the coronary care unit staff band together to discuss alternatives for future policy, even if their talks are constructive, this action may well be viewed by the administration as an act of mutiny—with unfortunate consequences for both sides. It will be interesting to see if these scenarios change in the future as more nursing departments are becoming decentralized. For instance, on primary care nursing units the staff nurse has total responsibility for planning and delivering nursing care. This carries with it the authority for decision making and ultimately results in increased accountability. Thus the staff nurses begin to view nursing administration differently as they experience the support given for their nursing judgments.

The physician who does not consult a nurse about his patient misses the opportunity of staying several steps ahead in the care of that patient. Failure to consult with the nursing staff guarantees defective knowledge about a patient's total care. So, too, the nursing administration that fails to consult its staff about unit activities is condemned to plan with incomplete or even inaccurate knowledge of the situation. Usually the paranoia tends to be strongest when unit structure or personnel are changing. These are the times when communication should be increased and enhanced rather than discouraged. When the staff members say that they are not willing to give any thought to a problem because the decision will be made arbitrarily anyway, they are avoiding (and perhaps afraid of) a basic responsibility. Staff members seldom expect or want democracy in the administration of a unit, but interpersonal relationships and morale will be vastly improved when they believe their opinions and work are recognized and respected.

While running a unit democratically is initially threatening to staff and always takes more time to reach decisions, the rewards are worthwhile. The unit truly becomes the staff. There is active participation by all. Staff members begin to run their own staff meetings in the absence of the head nurse and update her on topics discussed.

Nursing hopelessly failing hearts

It has been said that the only certainty in caring for the terminal coronary patient is that no one wants a patient to die on his or her shift. Balloon- or pressor-dependent patients cannot live forever, and when the imminence of death becomes evident, arranging for humane terminal care is an arduous task. We have witnessed a change in this attitude as demonstrated by the following example. Ms. B., a 67-year-old woman with idiopathic hypertrophic subaortic stenosis, had been transferred from another hospital. After suffering a myocardial infarction, her care consisted of intubation and the intra-aortic balloon pump. Weaning

Ms. B. from the pump was simple compared with the problems encountered weaning her from the respirator. A tracheostomy was eventually performed. Ms. B. remained in the coronary care unit for 3 months, courageously fighting off one complication after another. During that time every staff member had at least assisted in her care or cared for her directly. The entire staff had developed close feelings for Ms. B. Finally, the day came when Ms. B. was to have surgery (myectomy). She was prepared and so were her caretakers. Five minutes before Ms. B. was to be placed on call for the operating room, she sustained a respiratory arrest. Status epilepticus persisted for over 16 hours and was finally suppressed by heavy sedation. After that period, Ms. B. was unresponsive although sedation was lifted. The staff was stunned. No one could understand the turn of events. When it became evident that Ms. B. would not recover, each staff person who cared for her was prepared for the death to occur on his or her shift to spare the rest of the staff the painful experience of watching Ms. B. linger. While there are not and never have been any pat answers or solutions to caring for the terminal cardiac patient, there are many pitfalls to be avoided.

Vague communication about treatment plans is probably the worst hazard. Even when it has been agreed that a patient is not to be resuscitated, the meaning of "do not resuscitate" (DNR) may not be specified. The interpretations are legion—"Shock him once," "Do everything except intubate," and "Call a code but walk to the phone" are typical examples. In this way responsibility is passed from the primary physician down the line, so that the real decision about resuscitation may be left with anxious house staff or nurses in the coronary care unit. When resuscitation measures are to be limited, the exact specifics must be spelled out in advance. Moreover, those who think that DNR simply means hands off know very little about terminal cardiac illness and nothing about caring for human beings. One day a house officer and a nurse complained because an elderly woman who had been brought into the emergency room with acute pulmonary edema had been treated vigorously and brought to the coronary care unit. A nurse summed it up perfectly: "That's not a very pleasant way to die." Naturally, allowing acute pulmonary edema to go untreated in a conscious person would be an act of cruelty, not humanity. So too, efforts to ensure the greatest possible comfort for a terminally ill patient usually require keen foresight and detailed daily discussions of that individual's personal needs.

Additional forms of conflict complicate this matter further. The private physician may insist on prolonging life unnecessarily, not because it is appropriate but out of resentment for nurses and house staff who have been pushing for a treatment designation of "comfort measures only." In such a case patient care becomes an authority struggle. In one case the nurses were complaining bitterly about the treatment orders written for a 62-year-old woman with end-stage congestive heart failure. One nurse expressed anger because even though the patient had been specified as DNR, she was maintained on 2 micrograms of levarterenol bitartrate (Levophed) per minute. "That's totally inconsistent. How can a person be DNR and be getting Levophed?" When asked what happened when the medication was discontinued, the nurse replied that the patient developed pulmonary edema. The staff did not want the patient to die in this way, and further discussion revealed how strongly the staff disliked this woman. She was indeed a troublesome, complaining, demanding person. Her family also found it difficult to tolerate her. Orders for her care had specified DNR for about 10 days. When one of the nurses asked how long the situation was going to continue, it became clear that everyone had a feeling of impatience. When would the patient have the "courtesy" to make her exit? In this case communication had been excellent, but the patient was not "cooperating" with the treatment plan. Moreover, she continued to be herself and, as throughout her life, she was a difficult person to relate to. It is important to acknowledge embarrassing realizations such as wanting a troublesome patient to die and get it over with. Such responses are spontaneous and normal, but they can never be made the basis for treatment recommendations. If acknowledged, it is possible to talk about the real problem—caring for a person with abrasive traits—instead of the sham problem that the patient's life is being needlessly and inhumanely prolonged. In Massachusetts, the Dinnerstein 5 decision has allowed and encouraged the physician to write in the chart specifically how a terminally ill patient is to be treated when death is imminent. This has helped to clear some of the confusion surrounding DNR orders. Nurses and physicians are more willing to communicate openly regarding DNR measures.

It is more complicated and probably more difficult to provide for the terminal cardiac patient than for the terminal cancer patient. Pressors, antiarrhythmics, phlebotomies, pacemakers, and other procedures may be required to accomplish this. Moreover, the treatment may require modification from day to day. If the patient unexpectedly begins to recover, clearly the order DNR needs to be specifically reclarified. If there is not daily communication between physicians and nurses about both the treatment procedures and their rationale and justification, conflict is guaranteed. Where communication is already poor and mutual distrust is high, no reasons will be given by the physicians and no questions will be asked by the nurses. When a nurse is feeling unappreciated by the staff physicians, she is likely to absent herself from rounds, either in body or in mind. A complaint that is often heard concerns a patient's Swann-Ganz and arterial lines that have been left in needlessly, causing unwarranted distress. The reasons for leaving them in had been discussed and clarified on rounds. Why this was either unheard or uncommunicated usually had more to do with the emotional climate of the unit than the failure of a notetaking system or the mechanics of giving a report.

Caring for patients suffering from terminal congestive heart failure or electrical instability is an impossible task. A psychiatrist who was asked to see a coronary care unit patient with terminal congestive heart failure spoke with the patient and returned to the nursing station visibly irritated. "Ten years ago I was called here to see a patient with terminal congestive heart failure and now, ten years later, you people still don't know how to take care of them!" This of course was a massive projection that he himself hadn't learned anything in 10 years—as though miracles happen. There simply is no way of caring for desperately ill people without undergoing a considerable amount of distress, uncertainty, self-doubt, and the wish to be elsewhere. A reasonable first step is to acknowledge that the terminally failing ventricle of a conscious person poses a problem that will tax the technological ingenuity and empathic virtues of every person who becomes involved.

What can be done about this problem? Because heavy burdens are lighter when shared, the group process can again be extremely helpful in analyzing terminal situations, so that the response of the team can be unified and at full strength. The problem of caring for one patient in his early forties is an example. This patient had inoperable coronary artery disease and was dependent on an intra-aortic balloon catheter. The staff's feelings toward him were basically negative. A person who communicated mostly by grunts, he showed little response except irritation to those in his environment. One of the nurses began a group meeting by saying she found herself hoping not to be assigned to take care of him. A quick survey revealed that if the man had redeeming features that made communication easier, no one had yet discovered them. On the other hand, feelings toward his wife and daughter were uniformly positive; in fact, the nurses also wondered how these two were able to tolerate their visits. The focus of treatment was therefore deliberately changed from trying to get the patient to communicate to making it easier and more pleasant for his wife and daughter to be in his room. Because the latter were communicative and responsive, this goal was quickly reached and the results were also quite helpful to the patient who clearly seemed more content when his family was present. Through his wife and daughter the nurses learned to know the patient somewhat better, and he, perhaps with less pressure and expectation to communicate, also seemed more appreciative.

It has been said that modern cardiology and cardiac surgery can work miracles. When we see many patients brought back from the brink of death by defibrillation and pacing, the intra-aortic balloon catheter, bypass procedures, and aneurysmectomy, it is hard to disagree. Perhaps it is an even greater miracle that a group of people can actually stand by to maintain the comfort of a person whose life they cannot save.

GENERAL PERSPECTIVES

The greatest enemy of coronary care unit morale is staff divisiveness. In studying morale scores of a coronary care unit staff under varying conditions of stress, it was learned that those conflicts stemming from the patient's condition could be handled without any measurable harm to the sense of harmony felt by the staff.[1] In fact, in many cases morale rose as demands of care increased. However, if the stress is generated within and among the staff, particularly by competitive jealousies over competence, the effects on group harmony are disastrous. A coronary care unit staff can face impending doom and tragedy and struggle with impossible tasks consistently only if staff members take their collective responsibility seriously. Ideally, learning to deal with group problems selectively is best accomplished through weekly group meetings. Any skilled group leader—nurse, psychiatrist, psychologist, social worker, or chaplain—who is willing to learn about the coronary care unit and its patients can be a helpful resource. Hopefully the methods developed in these meetings will be transferred so that every report presents an opportunity for one shift to enlighten, encourage, and support the other in an ongoing effort to improve the care of the most difficult and complicated patients. This will foster an effort to share rather than hoard knowledge and skill, so that open communication can simplify what suspicion, silence, and wounded pride make intolerable. In such an atmosphere, the patients will benefit and the staff will grow as well.

• • •

What elements in our personalities have led us to seek work in a coronary care unit? Are intensive care nurses a different breed from those who care for patients suffering in other parts of the hospital? At Duke University Medical Center, Gentry et al.[7] compared nurses working in the coronary care and other hospital units on measurements of depression, hostility and guilt, self-esteem, anxiety, general personality pattern, and level of job satisfaction. They found no differences between the two groups in general personality pattern, guilt, and self-esteem. But coronary care unit nurses appear to report more depression, hostility, and anxiety. These differences tended to be more pronounced among the Duke University Medical Center coronary care unit nurses than among those who worked in such a unit at the local Veterans Administration hospital. Gentry et al.[7] concluded that the key factors in determining differential responses were situational stresses such as overwhelming work loads, too much responsibility, poor nurse-doctor communication, cramped working space, and inadequate programs for continuing education. Again they emphasized the need to promote team pride and group spirit in situations characterized by extreme pressures.

On the other hand, it would be shortsighted to overlook the fact that these pressures also served to attract many of us to intensive care settings. Many of us like the work because the pace is fast, the level of tension is high, and the working conditions are such as to necessitate standing eye to eye with pain, delirium, death, and the challenge of doing the impossible. Paradoxically, the source of the greatest stress and of the greatest satisfaction is the same: caring for desperately ill patients. It is at once the hazard and the honor of the coronary care unit nurse.

However, in the midst of all the excitement, it is possible to focus on intensity itself to the exclusion of the development of responsible and responsive relationships. The pace alone, not the people, may be the stimulant. Occasionally a nurse has said that a rapid pace is preferable because it minimizes interpersonal contact. We all need to develop the capacity for intimate adult relationships. When sheer intensity replaces such relationships, this constitutes a bogus closeness and there is trouble. Increasing mechanical efficiency can become an escape from relating in more mature ways.

The coronary care unit can reveal humanity at its best and at its worst, and this applies as much to the staff as to the patients. We who work there put our own lives at risk in these settings—our own dignity, self-esteem, and self-respect. Failure to take the risk can be dehumanizing to ourselves or our patients. Because such a challenge is too great to be borne alone, the staff must share it collectively, with a devotion to one another that adequately reflects our dedication to our patients.

REFERENCES

1. Cassem, N. H.: What is behind our masks? A. O. R. N. J. **20:**79, 1974.
2. Cassem, N. H., and Hackett, T. P.: Sources of tension for the CCU nurse, Am. J. Nurs. **72:**1426, 1972.
3. Cassem, N. H., et al.: Reactions of coronary patients to the CCU nurse, Am. J. Nurs. **70:**319, 1970.
4. del Bueno, D. J.: Patient education: planning for success, J. Nurs. Admin. **8:**3-7, 1978.
5. Dinnerstein, S.: In the manner of Shirley Dinnerstein, Mass. App. Adv. Sc. 736, 747, n. 10, 1978.
6. Ferrigan, M.: New nursing horizon: the cardiac nursing specialist, Int. Nurs. Rev. **13:**19, 1966.
7. Gentry, W. D., Foster, S. B., and Froehling, S.: Psychologic response to situational stress in intensive and nonintensive nursing, Heart Lung **1:**793, 1972.
8. Nelson, K.: C.P.R. training for families of cardiac patients: one approach to the problem of sudden death, Unpublished Master's thesis, Boston College, 1977.
9. Pentecost, B. L., et al.: Organization of a coronary care unit in a general hospital, Br. Med. J. **3:**298, 1967.
10. Pozen, M., et al.: A nurse rehabilitator's impact on patients with M.I., Med. Care **XV:** 830, 1977.
11. Price, T. R., and Bergen, B. J.: The relationship to death as a source of stress on a coronary care unit, Omega **8:**229-238, 1977.
12. Simon, N. M., and Whitely, S.: Psychiatric consultation with MICU nurses: the consultation conference as a working group, Heart Lung **6:**497-504, 1977.
13. Storlie, F.: Patient teaching in critical care, New York, 1975, Appleton-Century-Crofts.
14. Woodwark, G. M., and Gauthier, M. R.: Hospital education program following myocardial infarction, Can. Med. Assoc. J. **106:**665, 1972.

SECTION THREE

REHABILITATION

7

Psychological aftermaths of myocardial infarction

A. DALE GULLEDGE

The animal's heart is the basis of its life . . . the sun of its microcosm; on the heart all its activity depends, from the heart all its liveliness and strength arise.

WILLIAM HARVEY, 1628

Despite shorter periods of hospitalization and earlier permission to return to work,[32,45,84] evidence indicates many patients are reluctant to return to work following a myocardial infarction.* Wynn[90] documented that if proper psychosocial management had been provided during and following the heart attack, unemployment 6 months later probably could have been averted. He also found that in approximately half of his 400 patients there was *unnecessary* emotional distress. Wishnie et al.[89] reported that at 6 months to 1 year after a heart attack, 88% of their patients were still either anxious or depressed, 55% had sleep disturbances, 38% had not returned to work for psychological reasons, and 83% complained of weakness. In *all* of the patients' families there was evidence of significant emotional conflicts subsequent to the heart attack, 75% of the problems being the result of "differences over medical instructions for convalescence."[12]

In the Göteberg studies of more than 1000 patients, depression, anxiety, irritability, and exhaustion were noted at least 3 months after myocardial infarction, and these symptoms were appreciably more frequent than in the control population.[2,78,86] Klein et al.[48] concluded that features of "invalidism" usually began early in the convalescent experiences of the patient with myocardial infarction. They suggested early identification and treatment of anxiety, fear, or depression were important for the postcoronary patient. Furthermore, they emphasized that "the spouse should be included in an open discussion of the meaning of

*See Goble et al.,[26] Groden,[31] Klein et al.,[48] Weinblatt et al.,[82] Wincott and Caud,[88] and Wynn.[90]

symptoms and any specific modifications of activities and roles.[48] Nagel et al.[59] found anxiety and depression in 55% of the patients still at home, and these symptoms were the most common noncardiac causes of persistant invalidism. In 52% of those patients who were not working, there was no clinical evidence of residual heart damage; Nagel et al. concluded that adverse emotional reactions were not dependent on the severity of the heart attack but seemed related to inadequate medical instructions about fitness and work or how to prepare for the resumption of normal activities.[59] There is increasing evidence to indicate that failure to recognize, prevent, and treat the psychological or psychosocial concomitants of a myocardial infarction leaves a situation fertile for the development, at times, of serious psychological problems. Furthermore, minimal benefit seems to accrue to the patient if his life is saved by elaborate hospital care but he is then returned to environmental conditions in which he feels he cannot function.

This chapter, then, is a review of some of the common problems that affect the patient after his heart attack, with solutions to return him more quickly to a happier life at home, work, and play.

PATIENTS' EMOTIONAL REACTIONS

Although the patient who has had coronary thrombosis may have experienced the usual anxiety and depression while in the coronary care unit,[12] many such patients after leaving the hospital have yet to feel and comprehend the complete effects of their illness.[41,49,52,69] As Jenkins has shown in Chapter 1, prior to myocardial infarction many of these patients are ambitious, aggressive, impatient people, excessively dedicated to work, who often labored long without much personal satisfaction.[24,46,55] Yet these are the same people who initially (often unwillingly) must be at home all day, faced with problems of home routines, dealing with an oversolicitous, anxious spouse, and trying to cope with the noise and conflicts of their children. In view of these domestic problems together with the multitude of instructions regarding medicine, diet, and physical activities and the patient's attempts to adjust to his own ongoing reactions to the ramifications of a heart attack that is affecting his work, income, and social relationships, it is not surprising that confusion frequently envelops both the patient and family and that emotional problems ensue.

Croog et al.[17] have commented on the stages of recovery associated with heart attacks, yet there is no agreement as to what approaches are appropriate at any given stage.[10,50,85] Despite many studies, part of the problem in identifying temporal events and emotional issues still remains the failure of the physician or nurse to recognize such emotional problems as anxiety or depression in the postcoronary patient,[52] either because *time has not been taken* to identify the psychological problems or because the training, sensitivity, or interest to identify emotional issues is lacking. During the first months at home, anxiety,[48,89,90] depression,* weakness,[71,89] fear of sexual arousal,[15,90] and disturbed sleep[15,90] are common. The patient frequently fears death, pain, dyspnea, and further heart attacks and he is not infrequently irritable or nervous, yet he tends to avoid complaining about such problems during subsequent office visits; these problems are usually uncovered *only if the patient is directly and specifically questioned about what bothers him.*[89]

If those around the patient prevent him from working through normal emotional processes in response to a crisis, the normal reactions of disbelief, anger, denial, or depression may persist or intensify. Such unresolved processes may prevent the patient from accepting his condition and maladaptive problems may ensue, especially if before the myocardial infarction the patient had difficulty in adapting to life stresses.[9,64-67]

One common type of maladaptive behavior occurs in the counterphobic denier who ignores medical recommendations concerning his physical activity, work, diet, medication, and sex. In extreme instances, this "supermale" image leads to a disregard of symptoms and the development of a serious self-destructive pattern. Often this type of behavior is observed in the patient who continues to smoke, fails to keep an appointment, disregards the importance of medications, and continues to overindulge in physical activity, all the while verbally and nonverbally discounting medical suggestions. Although some patients with heart disease may be less willing to accept their illness as compared with other types of patients,[18,29,52] certainly patients who manifest this type of extreme maladaptation, who dismiss logic and ignore medical advice as they attempt to cope with their underlying emotional concerns, will need more than the usual care. As Olin and Hackett[60] have noted, "One cannot help but wonder, on the basis of this study, how many patients die simply because they have no one available to correct the flaw, created by denial, in their perception of reality."

Another common maladaption is that of the excessively helpless and dependent person who becomes a "cardiac invalid." If excessive deconditioning is allowed to develop as a result of overrestricting activity and if physician, family, or friends permit overprotective attitudes, unchecked, excessive somatic preoccupations may ensue. As with all significant physical inactivity, the normal sequels to deconditioning consist of tachycardia, orthostatic hypotension, shortness of breath, and weakness[83,84]—symptoms that can be interpreted by the patient and taken as "proof" of cardiac impairment. Such a patient comes to expect others to take care of him, and his heart becomes the principal basis of his relationships with those in his environment as he extracts the desired emotional gains socially, economically, and vocationally. The physician must be on the alert for such patients because unnecessary medication or hospitalization and unwarranted

*See Cay et al.,[14] Crawshaw,[15] Hellerstein,[36] Wishnie et al.,[89] and Wynn.[90]

probing into heart function confirm such a patient's fears about his physical condition and may delay his return to realistic levels of physical and emotional functioning and responsibility.[36,43]

Depression can be successfully prevented or treated if several concepts are kept in mind. Nonspecific, vague, or generalized statements should be stringently avoided to reduce confusion and conflicts between patient and spouse.[12,28,48] Letting the patient know specifically about his medical progress helps reduce anxiety and fosters hope. As the patient begins to develop trust, he usually is able to better ventilate his feelings because he learns to know what to expect and what is "normal" in his rehabilitation; this in turn enhances the working through of his grief concerning the loss of his "old self," or as Cassem and Hackett[12] put it, "the healing of an ego infarct." A specific, progressive program of physical activity is critical[83,84] and should be based on the program previously prescribed in the hospital.[12] The details of this program are usually best determined by appropriately controlled stress-exercise testing and telemetric monitoring.[7,70,76] As both the patient and spouse begin to feel secure about the levels of physical activity based on features such as pulse rate or better recognition of physical or emotional fatigue, the patient begins to realize he has not necessarily lost control over his physical or emotional destiny, and his self-esteem begins to return while his depression declines.

Attention should be directed toward the temporal relations between life-style and cardiac risk factors,[27,44] so that the patient can begin to reevaluate himself and learn what exacerbates or causes physical or emotional stress. Usually this is accomplished by taking the necessary time and offering ample and useful information, being prepared to repeat many times the important issues relevant to the patient. With the systematic use of repetitive positive reinforcement, the patient gains a new sense of satisfaction as he acquires new restitutive approaches that allow him to cope. Understandable and rational behavior on the part of those in charge of his care, coupled with substantial genuine interest, enhances patient independence and decision-making ability and prevents unnecessary emotional problems such as depression—all this while personal growth is promoted.

SPOUSES OF POSTCORONARY PATIENTS

The importance of the family in the recovery of cardiac patients is not well recognized by many health care professionals. According to a World Health Organization report, even neurotic individuals can adjust to severe cardiac impairment if they are constantly integrated into a strong, supportive, reasonable, but not overprotective, healthy family structure, which accepts and understands the illness.[69] Regarding the patient's wife, Crawshaw has remarked as follows:

> It has been said that the patient may recover from his coronary but that his wife may not. She has often seen her husband when he looked near to death, she may have been warned

> that he could die. . . . She has the same fears, lack of knowledge, and misconceptions as her husband. . . . Months after the infarct many wives report that they lie awake listening to their husbands' breathing to make sure that he is still alive. . . . She may also collapse under the strain of anxiety, become sick, depressed, develop chest pains. . . . Alternatively, wives may take over decision-making and bread-winning roles and become highly overprotective; this may increase the patient's feelings of helplessness and despondency.*

In effect, a myocardial infarction has considerable influence on the spouse—usually the wife—and her reactions, capacities, and attitudes are generally critical in the patient's rehabilitation.

A frequently described reaction of the spouse to the patient's return home is oversolicitousness.† Although postcoronary patients may intellectually understand their spouse's behavior as a manifestation of concern, they often feel upset that close supervision has been "imposed" on them.[6] For example, if a wife insists on performing the most menial tasks for the patient, this may be her attempt to handle her own underlying anxiety fears of possible death or reinfarction in her mate.[89] Moreover, many wives who have lived with a work-driven, tension-addicted, aggressive man for years prior to the coronary event despair at being in the involved position of "again" trying to change their husband's approach to life. They assume it will be a struggle.

Commonly, wives feel better when their husbands leave the hospital but subsequently feel much stress because they suddenly feel bereft of understanding and support they often had when their husbands were hospitalized. Anxiety, depression, numerous psychosomatic symptoms (including chest pain and palpitations), and sleep and appetite disturbances are not uncommon.[1,17,75,89,90] In one study of British wives, 38% manifested considerable distress as their husbands recovered. Problems of dependency and irritability seemed to often combine to produce significant marital tension.[75]

Wives often feel in a dilemma over how to deal with their recuperating husbands.[44,68] If they show concern, they are accused of being punitive and overprotective, but if they limit their concern and attempt to avoid unnecessary helplessness in their husbands, they are considered unsympathetic. For difficult-to-manage patients—those who failed to modify high-risk behavior—Hoebel[44] recommends brief, outpatient interactional therapy with the spouse for modifying her methods of dealing with her husband, thus reducing her husband's high-risk behaviors. Although the study was small, in each instance when the wife made the prescribed changes in interacting with her husband, desirable alterations in one or more of his high-risk behaviors resulted. Many wives, despite careful hospital instructions, do not fully understand the purposes of diets or know how to

*From Crawshaw, J. E.: Community rehabilitation after acute myocardial infarction, Heart Lung **3**:258, 1974.

†See Adsett and Bruhn,[1] Bilodeau and Hackett,[6] Klein et al.,[48] Wishnie et al.,[89] and Wynn.[90]

prepare savory low-fat, low-salt meals.[68] If the other family members continue to eat in the same manner while the patient is struggling to lose weight, the wife is frequently accused of being "unsupportive."

Many wives believe they contributed to their husband's heart attack and subsequently attempt to inhibit the expression of strong feelings for fear of causing angina, infarction, or even death.[15,48,75,86] Wives may withdraw unless counseled to share with tact and sensitivity, their thoughts and feelings with their husbands. If she suppresses her concern and avoids open discussion with her husband, she may convey to him that he is not worth much, thereby intensifying his humiliation and depression. Because of misunderstandings about ischemic heart disease, misinterpretation of instructions, and lack of information on what is normal or what is to be expected, the wife is left ineffectual at times when she needs to respond to problems.[48,89]

As Wynn[87] has emphasized, wives may experience *unwarranted* distress. Unnecessary problems in the convalescent phase could probably be mitigated if, beginning in the hospital, the physician and nurse would prepare the wife for the usual home difficulties and plan to include the wife in follow-up visits with the physician with the goal of imparting information in a clear, usable form.

Routine outpatient groups are often an invaluable aid for the wife during her mate's recovery.[1,28,68] It gives her the necessary time to discuss her feelings openly, a process that allows for a cathartic effect. Specific educational information regarding the nature of heart disease can be presented; this will give a wife a better idea of what to expect of herself and her husband during the process of rehabilitation. "Unique" and "lonely" feelings are usually dissipated as a spouse learns that others in similar circumstances have experienced similar feelings and have managed to cope and function well. For many wives a group setting promotes a better assessment of reality and provides opportunities to act more appropriately as they analyze their roles and attitudes and decide how these may contribute to disorganization or tension in the home setting. In essence, the wife learns to realize that the recovery process is a time-limited, sequential process that involves different coping patterns at different phases of her husband's convalescence and that it is *dependent on specific information* as she learns to deal with her husband's feelings as well as her own.

SEXUAL PROBLEMS OF POSTCORONARY PATIENTS

After the fear of dying from a heart attack has passed, nagging anxieties and questions often arise concerning sex.[1,6,75] "Is sex safe?" "Should we stop if it causes pain?" "Will my heart attack make me impotent?" Answers to such questions involve many factors other than the degree of heart damage or the residual of angina. Previous physical conditioning, age, gender, patterns of sexual activity before the heart attack, and many other issues need to be considered as answers are provided for patient and spouse following a heart attack.

Since knowledge often prevents or attenuates uncertainty and fear, why have there been problems with sex in the postcoronary patient? The most common answer to the question is probably that sex is rarely openly considered and discussed. If the subject is discussed, medical opinions are often so vague that misconceptions remain concerning diminished libido,[75] fear of sudden death with coitus, impotence, angina with intercourse, and dyspnea.[39,40,79,81] Wives notice significant changes in sexual activity in themselves as well as the patient during the first 3 months after hospital discharge, these changes being attributed to "increased tension, anxiety, and irritability"[75] in both partners. Wives who previously enjoyed sexual activity attributed their husband's decline in sexual activity to their own anxiety about the *safety* of coitus. Of a group of men who had experienced a myocardial infarction 3 months or more previously, 42% experienced cardiovascular symptoms with coition.[40] Some of the basics to be considered and brought forward by the staff for sexual counseling of the patient and spouse should include specific facts about the physiological reactions of the heart to sexual activity.

With respect to the excitement, plateau, orgasmic, and resolution phases of coition,[58] angina or excessive tachycardia occurs most often in the resolution phase.[40] Peak heart rates in normal individuals usually occur with orgasm, as does peak systolic blood pressure.[22] Hellerstein and Friedman[39,40] found that middle-aged men recovering from a myocardial infarction experience short periods of cardiovascular stress (4 to 6 minutes) during rather short periods of sexual activity (10 to 16 minutes). Thus the *usual* demands of sexual activity approximate those of climbing two flights of stairs, walking briskly, or exercising in terms of 5 to 6 Mets.* This amount of work on the heart is well within the range of capability of 70% to 80% of the middle-aged men who recover from an uncomplicated myocardial infarction and go on to function at an exercise level of 8 to 9 Mets.[37] Moreover, arguments or driving in traffic often produce a greater risk of excessive tachycardia than sexual activity, and coition does not increase the heart rate significantly when compared with the individual's usual and routine occupational activities.[39,40] Thus for the majority of patients with an uncomplicated myocardial infarction, it can be anticipated that normal conjugal sexual activity is not beyond their residual energy capacities. What, then, are the potential problems?

Deconditioning symptoms produced by bed rest and inactivity rather than the infarction must be explained to patient and spouse as common processes. After

*One Met is the energy expended per kilogram of body weight per minute by a resting subject. One Met utilizes approximately 240 milliliters of oxygen per minute.

careful evaluation of the cardiovascular system, a prescribed progressive program of physical activity will enhance the efficiency of the patient's cardiovascular system and improve exercise tolerance.[37,40,83,84] Moreover, not only can the frequency and quality of intercourse be enhanced by reconditioning programs, but it can be anticipated that cardiac symptoms during coitus will become less frequent.[37] Certain body positions produce excessive isometric activity that in turn increases energy demands on the heart; if angina does occur with coitus, husband and wife should be advised about the different positions for intercourse that can often minimize cardiac work, pain, or unnecessary anxiety.[37,75] Clustering of physiological demands on the heart should be discussed; for example, coitus soon after excess fatigue, a heavy meal, drunkenness, or undue emotion should be avoided so that the patient can better use his cardiovascular system and avoid unnecessary demands on it.[30] Better control of symptoms and a return to customary sexual patterns enhance feelings of better self-esteem and often counteract depression.

Masturbation and extramarital intercourse also should be discussed with the patient in terms of excessive cardiac work and their avoidance during recovery from a myocardial infarction.[39,57] Impotence, diminished libido, and impaired ejaculation are often unexpected side effects of medications such as antihypertensives, major and minor tranquilizers, ganglion blocking agents, antidepressants, and hypnotics.[73] If such medications are producing bothersome sexual side effects, alternative regimens should be devised to prevent these unnecessary problems. Finally, overt or subclinical depression and anxiety should always be considered as possible causes for impaired libido or impotence and should be appropriately treated.[12,48,75,89] The patient or spouse should not assume that these are the physiological sequelae of a heart attack. If *specific* information is made available to the patient and spouse as to what can be safely demanded of a healing heart—and when and how—most sexual problems may well be prevented. With the combination of proper physical reconditioning, judicious use of medication, and avoidance of unnecessary physical or psychological stresses, most patients and spouses should be able to return to sexual satisfaction.

COMMON DRUG PROBLEMS

Qualitative measures, physical counting of medications, and interviews have documented clearly that patients often do not take their medications as prescribed.[11,56] Perlman et al.[63] observed that one fourth to one half of their patients did not take their medications after being discharged from the hospital after treatment of congestive heart failure. Of the patients at the Marquette Cardiac Work Classification Unit, 75% misunderstood their treatment recommendations.[42] Drug misuse often is not recognized as such by the patient; furthermore, it may be perpetuated by well-meaning but misguided friends and family (and at times even by health care professionals) who do not take into consideration the financial, pharmacological, or psychological needs of the patient. The problem then becomes one of identifying the reasons for drug noncompliance and taking appropriate steps to rectify the problem.

Economic factors

Older patients spend almost three times more money for drugs than do younger patients,[80] yet often they have less money to live on, and it is not uncommon to hear a patient say, "I can't afford to take medications, Doctor." Often a limited supply of medications is given to the patient with prescriptions, but these may never be filled because the patient does not have the money to pay for them. Occasionally, a patient may lack the money even to pay for transportation to purchase his medications. It is therefore always worth the time to assess the patient's insurance and financial status so that he is not left with a number of prescriptions for which he cannot pay. Drugs prescribed by generic rather than trade names often are cheaper. Drug samples are frequently available at different community agencies, but the patient has to be tactfully steered toward these resources.

Instructions for drug use

Almost all studies have indicated that the more numerous the medications, the higher the noncompliance rate.[5,19] This finding may be related in part to inadequate education and instruction of patient and family. Thus if drug regimens are to provide the greatest benefit with the least chance of morbidity, the patient and family need to understand *how* medications are to be taken. It is helpful if medication instructions for the patient and spouse are started *several days* before discharge from the hospital and if they are presented in a relaxed manner, allowing time for discussion, thought, and receptivity. If the instructions are not given until the day before or the day of discharge, the patient and spouse are often too anxious about going home to listen carefully. Patients and spouses need to be instructed about "borrowing" other people's prescriptions for similar symptoms, the dangers of over-the-counter drugs, and the potential problem of drug interactions (both of those prescribed and those bought over the counter).[34,51] The purposes of each medication must be presented explicitly and in terms that both patient and family can understand; the explanation should include detailed instructions on how each medication is to be stored, how long it is to be taken, how it is to be used (whether it is to be chewed, diluted in juice, and so forth), what the maximum daily dose is, and examples of the common possible side effects, such as dry mouth or light-headedness.

Psychosocial factors

Psychological problems may range from denial of the need for medicine to the confidence of the hypocondriac that it is absolutely essential to his existence. Dependence on hypnotics, laxatives, sedatives, analgesics, and tranquilizers must always be kept in mind as a potential problem for the type of patient who may become regressive, dependent, and depressed. For such a patient, drug dependency may often begin in the coronary care unit, as the milieu reinforces the need for medicine because of a "sick heart"; the medicine then becomes the means by which the patient continues to prove that he is sick and helpless, promoting the expectation that others are to be responsible for him. On the other hand, maladaptive denial[18] may make the patient excessively counterdependent or counterphobic, providing a justification for his refusal of medications. These patients require much patience from those responsible for their care while they are learning to accept the reality of their limitations and symptoms so that they may use their medications better.

Errors in taking medicines can be related to sociological factors; for example, the patient may live alone. One study[72] has shown that 42% of patients who lived alone used medications improperly as compared with 18% of those who lived with at least one other person. Since many of those who live alone are older people, factors such as eyesight, memory, judgment, daily habits, and ease of body movement become critical in effective planning for the use of medication.

USE OF COMMUNITY AGENCIES FOR POSTCORONARY PATIENTS

One study of patients with coronary disease indicated that on discharge from the hospital after a heart attack, 42% of such patients had some difficulty in adjusting.[13,14] This finding suggests that for many patients, social agencies might be frequently helpful in rehabilitation.[33] Yet when patients in one study were asked whether they had received any type of professional assistance in their adjustment after a heart attack, 68% reported that they had had no contact with any agency other than the doctor or hospital.[16] *Only 1%* indicated that their physicians had given advice about agencies or organizations that might help in altering or changing jobs, and only 2% replied that they had received any advice about agencies through which financial aid might be obtained.[16]

One study[14] demonstrated that only 33% of the patients after their first heart attack said they were working as hard as before their heart attack 4 months previously; 45% of those who were anxious or depressed complained of serious difficulty in returning to work 1 year later. It therefore seems important to identify as early as possible those patients to whom ancillary services or agencies might be most valuable. These patients can be identified early because it is possible to recognize patients who will need psychosocial help even within the first 7 to 10 days of hospitalization. These are primarily young people who tend to be anxious or depressed and who have histories of difficulty in coping. They often foresee difficulties in work, have financial or family worries, and are skilled, semiskilled, or unskilled workers.[14,16] Although the return to work, the quality of their work, and the continuation of employment are important, these are not the only rehabilitative goals and certainly represent only part of an individual's attempt to return to a satisfying life. Self-esteem, daily coping, acceptance of physical and psychological limitations, home physical therapy, aid in preparing meals, arranging transportation, help with medications, homemaker services, nursery school, and family counseling are only some of the important areas in which a variety of agencies might give assistance. Undoubtedly, systematic studies are needed to determine the ultimate effects of community agencies on the rehabilitative process,[53] but until such agencies are better utilized, the impact and exact roles of community organizations remain to be elucidated. Gelfand et al. summarized this problem well when they reported that "There is so much knowledge that is not now applied or that is insufficiently developed that millions of cardiovascular patients do not obtain the help that could be given."[25] Empirical data indicate that if physicians would consider the use of appropriate agencies early in their plan for care, at least some of the many problems of work and other key areas could be diminished or prevented.[13,14,16]

PHYSICIAN, PATIENT, AND THE OUTCOME OF REHABILITATION

The physician, as Balint[3] has said, "should prescribe himself in generous doses." But his effect can be either therapeutic or noxious. If his effect on his patient's recovery is therapeutic, it will be through his human traits; his concern, understanding, warmth, perceptiveness, and kindness may accomplish as much for his patient as his skill and knowledge.[8]

The role of the physician in predicting and determining the success of rehabilitation is enormous.[36,54,87] As Croog and Levine have noted, ". . . it would appear . . . that the physician's judgment, based on clinical knowledge, [is] probably a more useful predictor than the other variables tested."[16] In essence, the physician determines the programs that affect the future life of the patient and his family. For example, if the physician is unaware of contemporary concepts of cardiac rehabilitation or insists that he alone can determine the requisite needs of his patient, iatrogenic disease may ensue.[36] On the other hand, if he makes use of the collaborative skills of other professions, minimizes deconditioning, and advocates a return to work and the involvement of appropriate community agency resources, a comprehensive, individualized program can be devised to provide for the social, medical, and emotional needs of his patient and family.[28,36,77,83,84]

Taking time to talk and listen to the patient seems mundane, but often the patient or spouse curtails communications because the physician is "too busy to be bothered with our little worries," setting a fertile stage for possible future communication gaps.[23] It is essential that the physician take the time to *discuss* repeatedly with both patient and spouse the rationale for physical, emotional, and drug treatments and the expected consequences of the illness as they might affect home, work, and play.

Patience remains a critical quality in a physician, especially if the patient is beset with many "risk factors" and continues to approach his cardiac problems in a counterphobic manner. This type of individual makes it difficult at times for the physician to restrain himself from expressing strong disapproval as a patient continues to abuse bar, bed, and board. It is easy to forget that a sought-after attitude or behavior change may be beyond the patient's or family's abilities at a given moment, and the physician must avoid the tendency to inappropriately exert retributive authoritarian pressure.

As several workers have observed,[38,47,48] the physician himself may be the cause of adjustment problems as his patient or his patient's family responds to his verbal and nonverbal cues. The good physician-patient relationship, on the other hand, is based on the strength and dependability of the physician, and his keenness can help the patient to repair defenses weakened by anxiety and depression; this is the *art of medicine,* and it should be practiced without apology. If the patient misperceives his situation, a thorough explanation can do much to correct the patient's misconceptions[4,20,74]; what the patient knows and what the doctor expects his patient to know often are inconsonant.[21] A definitive explanation by the physician to patient and family corrects misinformation, attenuates anxiety, and enhances the patient's adherence to the program.[20] The patterns of relationships depend on the sensitivity, practicality, intellect, and social awareness of the physician[62] and influence what can be understood and subsequently used; how well the patient complies with his regimen depends in part on how well he understands his doctor and how well the doctor understands his patient.

GENERAL CONSIDERATIONS

Cardiovascular rehabilitation is directed toward treatment of the *whole* patient and includes not only treatment of acute medical problems but also direction of the patient with regard to the socioeconomic aspects of his illness. Assessment allows the patient's *total* resources to be matched to the demands of home, work, and play. Such assessment includes a number of considerations: (1) the natural and unique history of the disease, which includes the prodromal, acute, and recovery phases; (2) the physical, social, vocational, avocational, and economic resources of the patient and spouse; (3) the patient's and spouse's limitations in these areas; (4) the current environmental demands and conditions that are appropriate to the vocational and avocational lives of the patient and spouse; and (5) the physiological capacities and reactions to a panorama of activities, which include exercise and stress.

The disease

Rehabilitation begins with the acute illness. Coronary care involves necessary routines, but care must still be individualized. Monitoring systems have permitted the abolition of needless restrictions and should minimize or prevent the problems associated with deconditioning. Thus with an uncomplicated myocardial infarction, initial cardiac rhythm monitoring eliminates the absolute need for bed rest and permits the patient to wash and feed himself; this, early on, provides the basis for a positive attitude for the future and reassures the patient that he can be active and independent.

Implicit in successful rehabilitation is the need for all of the members of the medical team to communicate satisfactorily, consistently, and appropriately. (The nonverbal cues and attitudes by those caring for the patient are well known to often convey more than the spoken word.) The physician, the nurse, the dietitian, and the physical therapist should all be informed and agree regarding the course of recovery and must convey information *understandably* to the patient and spouse. *Nothing* should be assumed or taken for granted from the time of the patient's admission to the coronary care unit until his discharge from the hospital. This approach prevents fright and insecurity and removes many substantial and unnecessary barriers to successful rehabilitation. The *individualized* program, both in the acute and subsequent rehabilitative phases, will determine activity programs and will consider such problems as pain patterns, fatigue, weakness, syncope, pulse rate responses, and cardiac rhythms with activity. Known risk factors such as smoking, obesity, personality traits, hypertension, and diabetes should be routinely identified and systematically treated by *all* the team treatment members in the most efficient and consistent manner possible.

Resources

The patient's history and physical and laboratory examinations usually permit identification of the physiological resources of the patient, but complete assessment should also include the patient's emotional, social, avocational, and vocational resources. Personality traits and structure, premorbid emotional health, and attitudes toward illness and work are critical areas to assess, and these can usually be ascertained if *time* is taken to talk with, *not just to,* the patient and spouse. The family's interpersonal relationships and attitudes, recent life situations, and goals need to be carefully examined as they relate to the patient's age, work, and economic status and how these influence his rehabilitation potentials. Vocational evaluation includes assessment of basic intellectual and cognitive capacities, educational background, training, and employment experiences to appropriately return or shift the patient to a satisfactory vocational status.

Issues surrounding workmen's compensation, disability benefits, premature retirement, and social security benefits that are unclear often need to be clarified.

Regardless of the uncertainty and vagueness of this area, it is an important issue that all of us must strive to understand better and thereby enhance the success of our patient's rehabilitation.

Energy expenditure and limitations

Exercise stress testing may be useful in an attempt to quantitate and specify the cardiac efficiency that can be maximized by exercise. However, it should be remembered that such testing may correlate poorly with what actually occurs on a job because of significant environmental stress involving such problems as supervision, peer relationships, ambient temperatures, and emotional stresses. Adequate job description by the patient *and employer,* production demands, shift work, and weather conditions are just a few of the issues that must be considered to effectively help the patient in his return to a meaningful vocational existence.

Energy costs during rest, recovery, and exercise need to be well known by all team members if the patient is to learn what is safe, healthy, and appropriate. Conditioning, deconditioning, and emotional stress need to be clearly identified for the patient and spouse so they will not fall into the trap of inactivity for fear of death or aggravating the disease.

The team approach

Some of the issues in approaching the problems of good rehabilitation for the person with coronary disease seem obvious. Even so, each involved professional needs to understand the important contributions that can be made by the other individual disciplines—hence the need for and the establishment of clear, flexible, progressive, and staged programs in such areas as nursing, physical medicine, dietetics, and emotional health. Moreover, once such programs are established they must then be *integrated* into a routine and individualized rehabilitation program for the patient and family that will transcend individual professional boundaries and disciplines and functionally incorporate the concept of the "team" approach. Team effectiveness requires that each individual must work to understand the other, take time to resolve problems, and be certain that he or she is acting in the best interests of the patient. It is understood that "programs" cannot be definitive; rather, they serve to furnish the touchstones for clear, effective, and ongoing treatment for the patient and family. The effort to clarify the puzzling and eliminate the unknown prevents confusion and discomfort; most important, it does not entangle the patient in inappropriate and unnecessary problems.

SUMMARY

The purpose of rehabilitative efforts is to guide the family and patient toward normal living following a myocardial infarction. To restore the coronary patient to a meaningful life, the physician will probably need to organize and use the talents and training of many other professionals. Rehabilitation begins with the diagnosis and treatment of the acute coronary patient and continues with careful concomitant evaluation of the emotional, vocational, physiological, and educational capacities of the patient and family. Recovery for the coronary patient fully embraces the concept of comprehensive health planning and includes preventive concepts as well as treatment concepts. Successful recovery depends on the efforts of a number of professional people who take the time to repeatedly present coherent and appropriately timed interpretations that are related to the patient's premorbid vocational, leisure, and family life. Attainment of these goals requires that the physical, material, and emotional aspects of the patient's life be carefully detailed. Recovery planning probably should not exceed the patient's or family's capacity to function and should be assessed in a sensitive, practical fashion; changes should not be imposed on a patient but should be made when the patient is capable of active participation. Early planning, discussion, and anticipation of usual reactions to a myocardial infarction promote understanding, compliance, and prevention of unnecessary problems. To know what is normal and when to expect it provides useful information for the patient and family. Impaired marital relationships, depression, anxiety, and physical weakness so commonly described during the recovery period should be greatly reduced in intensity and duration if effective education, rapport, communication, and planning are established with the patient and his family.

REFERENCES

1. Adsett, C. A., and Bruhn, J. G.: Short-term group psychotherapy for post-myocardial infarction patients and their wives, Can. Med. Assoc. J. **99:**577, 1968.
2. Ander, S., et al.: Psykosociala faktorer vid hjärtinfarkt, Lakartidningen **68:**3695, 1971.
3. Balint, M.: The doctor, his patient and the illness, ed. 2, New York, 1964, International Universities Press.
4. Bellak, L., and Haselkorn, F.: Psychological aspects of cardiac illness and rehabilitation, Soc. Casework **37:**483, 1956.
5. Bertin, R.: Patient compliance with prescribed drug therapy regimen, Paper presented at Clinical Pharmacy Seminar, University of Minnesota, February, 1972.
6. Bilodeau, C. B., and Hackett, T. P.: Issues raised in a group setting by patients recovering from myocardial infarction, Am. J. Psychiatry **128:**73, 1971.
7. Bjernulf, A., Boberg, J., and Froberg, S.: Physical training after myocardial infarction, Scand. J. Clin. Lab. Invest. **33:**173, 1974.
8. Braceland, F. J.: The coronary spectrum: psychiatric aspects, J. Rehabil. **32:**53, 1966.
9. Bruhn, J. G., Chandler, B., and Wolf, S.: A psychological study of survivors and nonsurvivors of myocardial infarction, Psychosom. Med. **31:**8, 1969.
10. Buchman, E. A.: Stages of illness and medical care, J. Health Hum. Behav. **6:**114, 1965.
11. Caron, H. S., and Roth, H. P.: Patients' cooperation with a medical regimen, J. A. M. A. **203:**922, 1968.
12. Cassem, N. H., and Hackett, T. P.: Psychological rehabilitation of myocardial infarction patients in the acute phase, Heart Lung **2:**382, 1973.
13. Cay, E. L., et al.: Psychological status during recovery from an acute heart attack, J. Psychosom. Res. **16:**425, 1972.
14. Cay, E. L., et al.: Return to work after a heart attack, J. Psychosom. Res. **17:**231, 1973.
15. Crawshaw, J. E.: Community rehabilitation after acute myocardial infarction, Heart Lung **3:**258, 1974.

16. Croog, S. H., and Levine, S.: After the heart attack: social aspects of rehabilitation, Med. Insight **5:**10, 1973.
17. Croog, S. H., Levine, S., and Lurie, Z.: The heart patient and the recovery process: a review of the directions of research on social and psychological factors, Soc. Sci. Med. **2:**111, 1968.
18. Croog, S. H., Shapiro, D. S., and Levine, S.: Denial among male heart patients: an empirical study, Psychosom. Med. **33:**385, 1971.
19. Curtis, E. B.: Medication errors made by patients, Nurs. Outlook **9:**290, 1961.
20. Durbin, E., and Goldwater, L. J.: Rehabilitation of the cardiac patient, G. P. **9:**43, 1954.
21. Eichenlaub, J. E.: Clichés that confuse the patient, Med. Econ. **34:**242, 1957.
22. Fox, C. A., and Fox, B.: A comparative study of coital physiology, with special reference to the sexual climax, J. Reprod. Fertil. **24:**319, 1971.
23. Francis, V., Korsch, B. M., and Morris, M. J.: Gaps in doctor-patient communication: patients' response to medical advice, N. Engl. J. Med. **280:**535, 1969.
24. Friedman, M., and Rosenman, R. H.: Association of specific overt behavior pattern with blood and cardiovascular findings, J.A.M.A. **169:**1286, 1959.
25. Gelfand, D., Acker, J. E., Jr., and Hellerstein, H. K.: Rehabilitation of patients with cardiovascular disease other than stroke: community services. In Andrus, E. C., and Maxwell, C. H., editors: The heart and circulation, vol. 2, Washington, D.C., 1965, Federation of American Societies for Experimental Biology.
26. Goble, A. J., Adey, G. M., and Bullen, J. F.: Rehabilitation of the cardiac patient, Med. J. Aust. **2:**975, 1963.
27. Gordon, T., Kannel, W. B., and McGee, D.: Death and coronary attacks in men after giving up cigarette smoking, Lancet **2:**1345-1348, 1974.
28. Granger, J. W.: Full recovery from myocardial infarction: psychosocial factors, Heart Lung **3:**600, 1974.
29. Gray, R. M., Reinhardt, A. M., and Ward, J. R.: Psychosocial factors involved in the rehabilitation of persons with cardiovascular diseases, Rehabil. Lit. **30:**354, 1969.
30. Griffith, G. C.: Sexuality and the cardiac patient, Heart Lung **2:**71, 1973.
31. Groden, B. M.: Return to work after myocardial infarction, Scott. Med. J. **12:**297, 1967.
32. Groden, B. M., Allison, A., and Shaw, G. B.: Management of myocardial infarction: the effect of early mobilisation, Scott. Med. J. **12:**435, 1967.
33. Hamlin, R. H.: The role of voluntary agencies in meeting the health needs of Americans, Ann. Am. Acad. Pol. Soc. Sci. **337:**93, 1961.
34. Hammel, M., and Johnson, K.: Patient education with the elderly . . . the need and challenge, Minn. Pharm. **90:**8, 1974.
35. Harvey, W.: The circulation of the blood and other writings, London, 1963, J. M. Dent & Sons.
36. Hellerstein, H. K.: Intereducation and reeducation in the rehabilitation of the cardiac patient, Am. Heart J. **58:**425, 1959.
37. Hellerstein, H. K.: Rehabilitation of the post-infarction patient, Hosp. Pract. **7:**45, 1972.
38. Hellerstein, H. K., and Ford, A. B.: Rehabilitation of the cardiac patient, J.A.M.A. **164:**225, 1957.
39. Hellerstein, H. K., and Friedman, E. H.: Sexual activity and the post-coronary patient, Med. Aspects Hum. Sex. **3:**70, 1969.
40. Hellerstein, H. K., and Friedman, E. H.: Sexual activity and the postcoronary patient, Arch. Intern. Med. **125:**987, 1970.
41. Hellerstein, H. K., and Goldston, E.: Rehabilitation of patients with heart disease, Postgrad. Med. **15:**265, 1954.
42. Hellmuth, G. A.: Employability of workers handicapped by certain diseases: a guide for employers and physicians, Arch. Environ. Health **17:**389, 1968.
43. Hinohara, S.: Psychological aspects in rehabilitation of coronary heart disease, Scand. J. Rehabil. Med. **2:**53, 1970.
44. Hoebel, F. C.: Brief family interactional therapy in the management of cardiac-related high-risk behaviors, J. Family Prac. **3:**613-618, 1976.
45. Hutter, A. M., Jr., et al.: Early hospital discharge after myocardial infarction, N. Engl. J. Med. **288:**1141, 1973.
46. Jenkins, C. D.: Psychological and social precursors of coronary disease, N. Engl. J. Med. **284:**244, 307, 1971.
47. Kahn, S.: Rehabilitation of the cardiac: introduction to the general problem, Am. J. Cardiol. **1:**365, 1958.
48. Klein, R. F., et al.: The physician and post-

myocardial infarction invalidism, J. A. M. A. **194:**143, 1965.
49. Kubie, L. S.: Cited by Kaufman, J. G., and Becker, M. C.: Rehabilitation of the patient with myocardial infarction, Geriatrics **10:** 355, 1955.
50. Kübler-Ross, E.: On death and dying, New York, 1969, Macmillan Inc.
51. Latidas, C. J., and Berry, C. C.: Misuse of prescription medications by outpatients, Drug Intell. Clin. Pharm. **3:**270, 1969.
52. Levenson, R. M., Rosenman, R. H., and Schwab, J. J.: A summary of a symposium on counseling the cardiac patient on work and sex, Ohio State Med. J. **66:**1003, 1970.
53. Levine, S., White, P. E., and Paul, B. D.: Community interorganizational problems in providing medical care and social services, Am. J. Public Health **53:**1183, 1963.
54. Levine, S. A.: Physician's fear: a deterrent to rehabilitation among cardiacs, Geriatrics **15:** 534, 1960.
55. Liljefors, I., and Rahe, R. H.: An identical twin study of psychosocial factors in coronary heart disease in Sweden, Psychosom. Med. **32:**523, 1970.
56. Marsh, W. W., and Perlman, L. V.: Understanding congestive heart failure and self-administration of digoxin, Geriatrics **27:**65, 1972.
57. Massie, E., et al.: Sudden death during coitus: fact or fiction? Med. Aspects Hum. Sex. **3:**22, 1969.
58. Masters, W. H., and Johnson, V. E.: Human sexual response, Boston, 1966, Little, Brown & Co.
59. Nagel, R., Gangola, R., and Picton-Robinson, I.: Factors influencing return to work after myocardial infarction, Lancet **2:**454, 1971.
60. Olin, H. S., and Hackett, T. P.: The denial of chest pain in 32 patients with acute myocardial infarction, J.A.M.A. **190:**977, 1964.
61. Orlando, I. J.: The dynamic nurse-patient relationship, New York, 1961, G. P. Putnam's Sons.
62. Ort, R. S., Ford, A. B., and Liske, R. E.: The doctor-patient relationship as described by physicians and medical students, J. Health Hum. Behav. **5:**25, 1964.
63. Perlman, L. V., et al.: Precipitation of congestive heart failure: social and emotional factors, Ann. Intern. Med. **75:**1, 1971.
64. Rahe, R. H., and Arthur, R. J.: Life-change patterns surrounding illness experience, J. Psychosom. Res. **11:**341, 1968.
65. Rahe, R. H., and Lind, E.: Psychosocial factors and sudden cardiac death: a pilot study, J. Psychosom. Res. **15:**19, 1971.
66. Rahe, R. H., and Paasikivi, J.: Psychosocial factors and myocardial infarction. II. An outpatient study in Sweden, J. Psychosom. Res. **15:**33, 1971.
67. Rahe, R. H., et al.: Subjects' recent life changes and coronary heart disease in Finland, Am. J. Psychiatry **130:**1222, 1973.
68. Rahe, R. H., et al.: Group therapy in the outpatient management of post-myocardial infarction patients, Psychiatry Med. **4:**77, 1973.
69. Rehabilitation of patients with cardiovascular diseases, WHO Tech. Rep. Ser. 1966.
70. Rothman, R. M.: A comprehensive cardiac rehabilitative program, Heart Lung **3:**578, 1974.
71. Ruskin, H. D., et al.: MMPI: comparison between patients with coronary heart disease and their spouses together with other demographic data, Scand. J. Rehabil. Med. **2:**99, 1970.
72. Schwartz, D., et al.: Medication errors made by elderly, chronically ill patients, Am. J. Public Health **52:**2018, 1962.
73. Serafetinides, E. A.: Assessing the sexual side effects of psychotropic drugs, Hosp. Physician **8:**58, 1972.
74. Sibley, J. C.: The post-hospital treatment of the patient with cardiac infarction, Appl. Ther. **7:**300, 1965.
75. Skelton, M., and Dominian, J.: Psychological stress in wives of patients with myocardial infarction, Br. Med. J. **2:**101, 1973.
76. Starke, H., and Eliot, R. S.: Assessment of available stress testing techniques (treadmill, bicycle ergometer, etc.), Contemp. Probl. Cardiol. **1:**335, 1974.
77. The coronary spectrum, J. Rehabil. **32:**entire issue, 1966.
78. Tibblin, G., Lindström, B., and Ander, S.: Emotions and heart disease, Ciba Found. Symp. **8:**321, 1972.
79. Tuttle, W. B., Cook, W. L., Jr., and Fitch, E.: Sexual behavior in postmyocardial infarction patients, Am. J. Cardiol. **13:**140, 1964.
80. United States Services and Mental Health Administration, Public Health Service: Working with older people: a guide to prac-

tice. II. Biological, psychological and sociological aspects of aging, Washington, D.C., 1970, U.S. Government Printing Office.

81. Veno, M.: The so-called coition death, Jap. J. Legal Med. **17:**330, 1963.
82. Weinblatt, E., et al.: Return to work and work status following first myocardial infarction, Am. J. Public Health **56:**169, 1966.
83. Wenger, N. K.: Coronary care: rehabilitation after myocardial infarction. New York, 1973, American Heart Association.
84. Wenger, N. K.: The early ambulation of patients after myocardial infarction, Cardiology **58:**1, 1973.
85. Whitehouse, F. A.: The utilization of human resources: a philosophic approach to rehabilitation, Dis. Chest **30:**606, 1956.
86. Wilhelmsen, L., Tibblin, G., and Werkö, L.: A primary preventive study in Gothenburg, Sweden, Prev. Med. **1:**153, 1972.
87. Williams, B., et al.: Cardiac rehabilitation: questionnaire survey of general practitioners, J. A. M. A. **165:**791, 1957.
88. Wincott, E. A., and Caud, F. I.: Return to work after myocardial infarction, Br. Med. J. **2:**1302, 1966.
89. Wishnie, H. A., Hackett, T. P., and Cassem, N. H.: Psychological hazards of convalescence following myocardial infarction, J.A.M.A. **215:**1292, 1971.
90. Wynn, A.: Unwarranted emotional distress in men with ischaemic heart disease (IHD), Med. J. Aust. **2:**847, 1967.

8

Vocational rehabilitation and the coronary patient

D. KENNETH MITCHELL

The return to work following a myocardial infarction (MI) is socially desirable and symbolically important.[8] Historically, the resumption of work activities for the coronary patient has been laden with unsystematic methods of prescribing the amount of work the patient is able to do. Likewise, the patient's emotional readiness for work activities has been a minor feature in vocational considerations. Philosophical, technical, and programmatic advances in the prescription of work levels for the coronary patient have occurred in the last 5 years. The employer, physician, and patient need not guess as to the appropriate levels of physical work that can be done. Work evaluation centers, systematic exercise stress test protocols, and graded exercise programs provide reliable information to the physician, employer, and patient for vocational decision making. These technological advances have improved one phase of the vocational rehabilitation process—the prescription of work activity in relation to the patient's cardiopulmonary functioning.

Hospital cardiac rehabilitation programs have been developed to increase the coronary patient's knowledge of the disease process, to aid the patient to cope emotionally, and to initiate a safe life-style following the myocardial infarction. Hospital cardiac rehabilitation programs are based on the concept of early mobilization and the systematic identification and modification of the patient's prominent physical and emotional risk factors. These programs are only now being systematically evaluated for their effectiveness in reducing the morbidity caused by myocardial infarction. Such programs generally involve a multidisciplinary approach that focuses on modifying risk factors such as obesity, smoking, type A behavior, and lack of exercise. Yet, efforts to aid the patient's vocational return and adjustment have not kept pace with available technology in risk factor reduction and work prescription. Therefore this chapter will not address the specific methods of prescribing work return, but will deal with the psychological ramifications of a myocardial infarction in relation to the conceptualization and delivery of vocational rehabilitation services to the coronary patient.

PROFILE OF VOCATIONAL PROBLEMS

Much of the inattention to work problems of the coronary patient is based on the perceived nonurgency of work issues in relation to the life-threatening events that exist during the early phases of coronary care. There is also an ongoing state of isolation that exists between medicine and industry. This isolation, even though industry and medicine are both concerned with the patient, creates poor communication concerning goals and expectations of the patient's coronary work activities. More importantly, in reaction to this isolation, the variability of problems exhibited and/or concealed by the coronary patient in an effort to return to work present a confusing picture for the rehabilitation specialist. In the patients' efforts to defend against or deny the implications of the myocardial infarction, they convince themselves and others that vocational rehabilitation services are not needed. This rationalization deters the delivery of timely and appropriate vocational rehabilitation efforts.

Philosophically, many employers, physicians, and patients believe that "the coronary patient" cannot or should not work at all. Present workmen's compensation and Social Security regulations pertaining to the coronary patient promote, within their definitions of disability and the attribution of the disease process, confusion in the evaluation of the disabilities levels. Such confusion in definitions generally creates disincentives to return to work and leads to a narrow conceptualization of vocational rehabilitation for the coronary patient. The above stated factors have created a vague picture of the type of overt and covert vocational problems that do, in fact, exist for the patient in his or her efforts to return to work.

Current studies indicate that a majority (65% to 75%) of the individuals experiencing an uncomplicated myocardial infarction attempt to return to work within 6 months.* An uncomplicated myocardial infarction is an infarction occurring without chronic arrhythmias, cardiogenic shock, or congestive heart failure. More specifically, it has been reported that approximately 40% of coronary patients attempt to return to work within 8 to 12 weeks after suffering an infarction. By 1 year following the myocardial infarction, approximately 85% to 95% of the coronary patients are reported to have returned to work.[30] In many of the reports of the patients' return to work, there is a variability of the patients' success rates in returning to work and in maintaining such work. This variability in the rate of return to work ranges from 40% to 95%. Follow-up studies suggest that initial success rates of patients returning to work are in the area of 80% to 85%. This

*See Cay,[6] Croog et al.,[8] Kushner et al.,[16] Mitchell,[22] and Muir.[25]

high percentage generally falls to 60% to 65% in 1-year follow-up studies.[16,25,30,35]

Research efforts have identified a variety of factors that preclude, delay, or enhance a successful return to work. Initially, the severity of myocardial damage provides one indicator of work return success. Nagle and Gargola[26] and Acker[1] indicated that severe cardiopathology is the major deterrent to work return. Obviously, the more medical complications from the infarction resulting in significant cardiopathology will provide less probability for the work return. Coupling factors such as advanced working age (55 years and over), premorbid heavy or stressful work load (emotional and physiological), sporadic work record, family instability, and lack of education about myocardial infarctions create significant reduction in the ability, opportunity, and/or desire for work.

The individual who experiences an uncomplicated myocardial infarction, does not possess obvious work traits that could create vocational problems, yet still has difficulty returning to work creates an enigma for the cardiologist, family physician, and employer. Research efforts have presented an array of factors that characterize those coronary patients who do not return to work, yet only have minimal myocardial damage. For example, Gelfand and Hagen[11] provided a classic picture of the individual who does not return to work following an uncomplicated myocardial infarction. They suggested that physical capacities were not sufficient to predict a work return. The patient's emotional response and attitudes toward the future differentiated between those who went back to work and those who did not. Those patients who were less depressed and had a positive outlook on life were more likely to return to work at levels appropriate for their functional capacities. Garrity[10] observed that patients with positive perceptions of health status, as well as a high degree of external locus of control, were more likely to return to work. This suggested that those individuals who relied on external forces in their environment to direct their behavior had a better probability of returning to work.

In a study of vocational rehabilitation activities of patients who experienced an uncomplicated myocardial infarction (NYHA Classification 2B), Mitchell[22] found multiple predictors for work return. This study pointed out several common activities within the person's daily life that provide an index as to the ongoing adaptation in the normalization process. It was observed that the length of time between the myocardial infarction and the resumption of hobbies discriminated between the working coronary patient and coronary patient who had not returned to work. The patients who eventually returned to work resumed their hobbies significantly earlier than those patients who had not returned to work. Likewise, the time between myocardial infarction and the resumption of sexual activities also discriminated between those patients who were working and those who were not. For those patients who were working, the resumption of sexual activities occurred significantly later in the rehabilitation process than for those patients who were not working.

Mitchell[22] also observed that the coronary patients who had returned to work had a high need for autonomy and introspection. Those patients who did not return to work did not have these particular characteristics. It was also observed that those patients with low need for change in their lives had a higher probability of returning to work. The implications for these findings are: (1) the group of patients who were identified as having mild myocardial infarction damage had a variety of work-related problems initiated by the heart attack and (2) major discriminators regarding work success were not of a physiological nature but were characterized by patients' need levels within their everyday activities. These findings suggested that a vocational counseling program should be of a very specific nature to identify the needs or need systems that may be directing individuals' behavior following the infarction. Therefore a systematic conceptualization of vocational rehabilitation must consider the variety of need levels that may facilitate work return possibilities.

Shiller and Baker[29] found that family stability, employment status at the time of the myocardial infarction, patient's emotional state, and the skill level of the individual's precoronary occupation were predictive of a work return. They elaborated that a stable family situation, regardless of whether or not the patient was married, promoted recuperation and eventual return to work. They also indicated that the vocational opportunities for the patient after the myocardial infarction were greatly enhanced when the patient was employed before the infarction. Vocational success was greater when the patient exhibited low levels of anxiety and depression during the recuperative period. It was also found that the patient's occupational level was predictive. That is, those individuals who were skilled laborers were more likely to return to work than those individuals performing unskilled work. This finding has been discussed in several other studies. For example, it has been observed that the patient's skill level or occupational characteristics, that is, blue-collar versus white-collar, significantly affected the rate of return to work, as well as the total number of coronary patients in that particular working group who returned to work. However, it has been observed that the blue-collar and white-collar workers eventually return to work in similar numbers, but the white-collar worker assumes a work role much sooner.[33]

Kushner et al.[16] observed in a controlled follow-up study of vocational activity of coronary patients that individuals who engaged in a 4-week, follow-up counseling program fared significantly better vocationally than those individuals who were not seen other than for medical follow-up. It was also found that patients who successfully returned to work had less physical disability, less exacting jobs before suffering an infarction, and a higher degree of emotional well-being than those who did not return to work. Those individuals who returned to work successfully did not consider their jobs a major cause of their illness.

The patient's explanation of the cause of a myocardial infarction is a factor that must also be considered in the rehabilitation process. As Kushner et al.[16] have indicated, those individuals who returned to work did not consider their jobs a cause of their illness. Legally, the explanation of the cause of myocardial infarction becomes important because it will direct the patient away from or toward a variety of activities that deal with compensation and potential litigation. Litigation within the rehabilitation process has been found to be a significant detractor for eventual vocational rehabilitation success.[7] Personally, the patient's explanation for the cause of the disability, regardless of the scientific explanation, may provide significant direction of the rehabilitation process. The patient's private explanation of the event may control future behavior in assessing the probability, method, and comfort in going back to work, as well as establish a "meaning" for the heart attack. This personal explanation must be assessed within the early phases of the rehabilitation process to detect the total impact the infarction may have on the individual. Individuals operating under significant misconceptions may not be able to utilize appropriate rehabilitation services.

In summary, the factors that delay or preclude a work return involve two major areas. Initially, the severity of myocardium damage coupled with factors such as advanced age, poor work history, heavy work load required after an infarction, and negative employer attitudes influenced the work return possibilities. Such factors preclude a positive work adjustment. These areas have been the traditional guidelines for predicting or prescribing work return and the application of vocational rehabilitation services. These characteristics are very obvious and must be attended to. Yet, these particular factors are only half the picture that leads to the success of the work return following the myocardial infarction.

The second group evolves from the current research that has provided the cardiac rehabilitation specialist with a profile of factors that give us a more comprehensive look at the elements of vocational rehabilitation success. As we have stated, factors such as chronic negative emotional response to the infarction, the patient's attribution of the infarction, the patient's sense of health and well-being after the infarction, and the patient's need levels have found to significantly discriminate between the patients who return to work and those who do not. Such factors suggest that the vocational return for the coronary patient does not happen automatically. Each case must be surveyed for potential saboteurs that are inherent in the significant emotional, psychological, and physical adaptations that are occurring constantly within the effort to return to work.

The return to work is accomplished by a majority of coronary patients. Yet this work return can be accomplished with a high degree of job and personal dissatisfaction.[3] This dissatisfaction, when not being dealt with in any systematic fashion, can be a deterrent to a quality life and can increase the overall stress on the patient. Such dissatisfaction, while generally not exhibited prior to returning to work, can be exacerbated once the person has returned to his old work environment. Heretofore, this dissatisfaction and emotional concerns have not been dealt with in any systematic way in follow-up services by cardiologist, family physician, or the employer. Identification of the psychological and interpersonal issues that exist prior to returning to work, but subsequent to the infarction, allow the rehabilitation specialist to develop the appropriate vocational rehabilitation services for the coronary patient.

CONCEPTUALIZATION OF VOCATIONAL REHABILITATION SERVICES

The vocational rehabilitation process for the coronary patient goes beyond the single event of physically returning to the job. The return to work, indeed, has very practical implications for economic and family stability, maintenance of the individual's self-esteem, and the continuation of the individual's vocational and economic development. More importantly, the work return, in many cases, is the symbol of successfully coping with the significant insult on the individual. Therefore, to deny the importance of vocational considerations in the person's life or to deal with them in a superficial way reduces the rehabilitation team's capacity to provide appropriate services.

The vocational rehabilitation process is a compilation of efforts by the patient, rehabilitation staff, and employer to facilitate the patient's work return and positive work adjustment. Within this process certain factors are critical. The patient's problem-solving skills, economic needs, emotional adjustment, and the commitment to return to work are as important as his cardiopulmonary functioning. Therefore, the conceptualization and delivery of vocational rehabilitation services must go beyond the simple matching of the work load on the job and the functional capacity of the coronary patient. Vocational rehabilitation services must also go beyond the retraining of the individual if the patient is unable to return to a particular job.

A contemporary view of vocational rehabilitation services is based on four principles, which provide a basis for developing an efficient and safe work resumption plan for the coronary patient. Each of the principles offers a specific component to vocational rehabilitation planning.

1. The myocardial infarction and subsequent coronary care process make an impact on the patient's total functioning.
2. Vocational rehabilitation planning must be a systematic process of problem identification and application of treatment strategies within critical adjustment phases of the recuperative period.
3. The myocardial infarction occurs within specific adult vocational developmental stages that determine the vocational meaning of the myocardial infarction.
4. Vocational rehabilitation services should be delivered by an interdisciplin-

ary cardiac rehabilitation team that appropriately links medical technology, emotional and social support, and industrial resources.

The first principle—*the myocardial infarction and subsequent coronary care process make an impact on the patient's total functioning*—pervades the entire process of rehabilitation. It has been readily observed that the myocardial infarction and the subsequent coronary care process not only affects the person physiologically but provides a significant insult to his psychological integrity.* This insult mobilizes significant emotional energies toward adaptation by the patient. In recent follow-up studies it is obvious that counseling makes a significant difference in the vocational potential for the individual.[16,30,35] Likewise, social support during the adaptation process immediately following the myocardial infarction and subsequent to discharge from the hospital allows individuals to systematically sort out emotional concerns that are related to vocational alternatives.[8,12] Reactions such as guilt, depression, and anxiety may pervade the whole rehabilitation process for the coronary patient. These reactions, coupled with the fear of death on increased exertion, can narrow the vocational and avocational life space of the individual. Such fears can disrupt the normalization process and create chronic invalidism.

While the patient is engaged in significant efforts to reduce the psychological impact of the coronary event, vocational concerns are many times a progenitor of anxiety in relation to economic stability and the perception of one's ability to be a productive individual. Social factors become prominent during rehabilitation in terms of interaction between the patient and spouse. Ibrahim et al.[14] point out very clearly that the relationship between the patient and the spouse is significantly affected by a myocardial infarction. Aldes et al.,[3] in a comprehensive review, corroborate Adsett and Bruhn's[2] work in that the spouse plays a significant component in the total adjustment process. Stress created within the family structure can have significant effects on the vocational possibilities and methods of returning to work.

Programmatically, this principle stresses the importance of early intervention and counseling. This counseling approach should be a broad-spectrum approach that deals with, not only personal issues, but the integration of personal and vocational issues as a natural component of rehabilitation programming.

The second principle—*vocational rehabilitation planning must be a systematic process of problem identification and application of counseling strategies within critical adjustment phases of the recuperative period*—operationalizes the concept of a total person approach in vocational rehabilitation planning. In any type of rehabilitation planning, it is mandatory that an accurate process of problem identification be carried out. Following appropriate problem identifica-

*See Aldes et al.,[3] Croog et al.,[9] Garriety,[10] Hackett and Cassem,[12] and Klein and Dean.[15]

tion, a systematic application of counseling and work return strategies can be performed.

With the complexities of the coronary patient's efforts to return to work, a broad-spectrum case conceptualization model is appropriate. Such a conceptualization must assess the patient's behavior, emotions, sensorium, thinking process, self-images, and social/vocational life-style. This assessment must be carried out within the context of the patient's adaptation within three critical periods following the myocardial infarction: (1) the patient's in-hospital activities (3 weeks postinfarction), (2) discharge and transition into his home (3 to 8 weeks postinfarction), and (3) long-term readjustment (at least 8 weeks).

Lazarus[18,19] has developed a multimodal counseling approach that identifies problems within specific modalities that can be treated with a variety of counseling approaches. This diagnostic and prescriptive counseling approach, while not specifically designed for the coronary patient, is highly applicable to the conceptualization of strengths and weaknesses in the coronary patient's repertoire of coping skills for work return. Lazarus[20] identifies the multimodal concept as a specific approach to assess the patient's functioning within seven primary modes: (1) behavior, (2) affect, (3) sensorium, (4) imagery, (5) cognitions, (6) interpersonal activities, and (7) drugs. Lazarus uses the acronym, *B.A.S.I.C. I.D.*, to guide the counselor in identification of positive and negative patient characteristics.

The B.A.S.I.C. I.D. encourages the counselor and patient to systematically identify, evaluate, and modify the single and/or interactive problems that may be sources of debilitation. Nieves[27] identifies the primary tenets of multimodal therapy as:

1. The individual is an acting, feeling, sensing, imagining, thinking, and relating human being.
2. The individual's different modalities are interactive in a psychological, behavioral, and biological sense.
3. Empirical observation and programmatic application of information directs therapist/client movement.
4. Therapy is an educational process to enhance the client's repertoire of effective coping responses.
5. Direct intervention in the "here and now" is based on social learning principles.
6. Counseling/intervention techniques or procedures to be used effectively resolve problems and are durable.
7. Total therapy covers the seven modes of B.A.S.I.C. I.D.

The multimodal process begins with an in-depth assessment of each model. The primary tools of assessment are the clinical interview, observation, and client report. For the coronary patient, the multimodal assessment procedure will in-

Table 8. Multimodal diagnostic prescriptive format treating the B.A.S.I.C. I.D.*

Modality	Assessment procedures	Sample	Sample treatments
Behavior	Behavioral analysis	Excesses; deficits; pattern	Assertiveness; physical exercise; behavioral contracting
Affect	Observation/ interview	Distortions; inappropriateness; absence	Systematic desensitization; role-playing; imagery tasks
Sensorium	Neurological assessment	Awareness; deficits nonawareness	Relaxation program; exercise program; surgical intervention
Imagery	Interview/imagery tasks	Self-images; ruminating fantasy; no images	Fantasy exercises; desensitization; blow-up technique
Cognitions	Interview/cognitive assessment procedures	Fallacious thinking; cognitive distortions; cognitive deficiency	Cognitive restructuring; rational emotive therapy; bibliotherapy
Interpersonal activities	Interview/ observation/ client-family report	Social withdrawal; secondary gains; decision-making problems	Role-playing; assertive training; cognitive restructuring
Drugs	Interview/ client-physician report	Nonadherence; abuse; nutritional deficits	Diet program; drug program; behavioral contracting

*This is a composite example of assessment procedures, problem types, and proposed treatments used in each modality, but not specifically for the problem stated.

clude procedures as ergometric stress testing, diet evaluation, standardized assessment of work values, job satisfaction, type A behavior assessment, and an on-site job analysis. The multimodal assessment efforts are designed to identify within the B.A.S.I.C. I.D. the (1) deficits, excesses, and ineffective patterns of behaving or coping, (2) affective states such as depression, anxiety, or lack of affect, (3) sensory distortions, neurological impairments, and somatic complaints, (4) self-concept, fantasy life, life images/dreams/symbolic representations, (5) fallacious thinking, and attentional distortions, (6) social awareness and maturity and interpersonal relations, and (7) drug/medication regimen, drug interaction, drug-induced behavior, and propensity to adhere to risk reduction programs.

On complete and total review of patient problems, the client and therapist utilize a diagnostic/prescriptive format (Table 8) to identify problems, prioritize needs, and select the effective treatment procedures within the counselor's clinical armamentarium. Significant efforts are made to identify the patient's receptivity to participate in the selected intervention strategies and to thoroughly explain the intervention procedures.

Counseling strategies that can be used in a broad-spectrum approach reflect a technical eclecticism in the application of cognitive/behavior modification techniques such as relaxation therapy, physical exercise programs, cognitive restructuring,[4] cardiac stress management problems,[31] self-instructional stress innoculation programs,[21] and multiple imagery procedures.[17] The multimodal conceptualization allows the counselor working with the coronary patient to identify the major factors that can enhance or sabotage specific rehabilitation efforts within the three critical phases. These problems can range from patient nonadherence to risk reduction programs, maintenance of exercise programs, fear of sexual activity, misconception of the disease process, and eventual work return adjustment.

The multimodal approach provides the cardiac rehabilitation specialist with the opportunity to clearly identify factors that enhance or reduce the patients' capacity to return to work. This type of case conceptualization couples the physiological, psychological, and social factors that lead to a positive work adjustment.

The first two principles provide the basis for developing appropriate rehabilitation programs for the coronary patient. The third principle—*the myocardial infarction occurs within specific adult vocational developmental stages*—determines the vocational meaning of the myocardial infarction. The vocational activity of the patient at the time of the infarction is a dynamic process combining age, work history, work and personal responsibility, needs, and aspirations. Obviously, vocational activities of each of the patients vary as to style and intensity. Such variations warrant specific assessment in relation to the patient's perception of the impact the myocardial infarction has on specific vocational development tasks the person is engaging in at the time of the infarction. A vocational developmental task is a "work or career task that arises at or about a certain period in the life of the individual." Successful achievement of this task will lead to the individual's happiness and success in later vocational tasks.[12] The interpretation or meaning of the infarction by the patient in relation to their vocational development is extremely important. This interpretation will direct the type and degree of vocational rehabilitation services needed or desired. The individual often sees the myocardial infarction as a barrier to his continued vocational development. Comments by patients indicate attitudes such as "things will never be the same," "I guess my goals will no longer be met," or "I'm not worth anything anymore." Other comments by clients suggest that their interpretation of the myocardial infarction has eliminated further growth as individuals and certainly narrows their career goals they may have within a company or a field of endeavor. Such comments should be taken as major influences on the person's perception of vocational alternatives. Specific vocational tasks that are prominent during the three decades of the highest frequency of myocardial infarction include advancement within the career, maintenance or stabilization of economic productivity, and consideration of eventual retirement activities. In many of the follow-up studies of coronary patients, the patient returns to work for 6 to 8 months and then for a variety of physical and emotional reasons decides to take an early retirement.[25,35] In many cases the decision to retire is based on the assessment by the patient that work is not as important as once thought and/or work is not worth the effort in relation to the perceived danger of incurring another infarction because of increased activity. Obviously, the continuation of the patient's vocational development has significant economic as well as personal ramifications.

The concept of secondary gains becomes increasingly prominent in the relationship between past vocational success, work return, and the coronary event. Secondary gains that arise from the myocardial infarction can be extremely subtle as well as dramatically obvious. In either case, secondary gains provide a variety of motivations to inappropriately return to or avoid work following the myocardial infarction. Secondary gains are those benefits derived from a disability or event that present a reason for participating in a socially unacceptable activity. For example, the patient may attempt to meet strong dependency needs by holding on to the sick role for a longer time than is desirable. Relationships with nurses and physicians or role changes with the spouse are examples of secondary gains. The patient may expect to be excluded from specific social or vocational responsibilities that would not be appropriate activities for a "coronary patient." Preinfarction vocational problems created by job dissatisfaction or vocational immaturity would provide the person with reason for not returning to a specific work site or a general state of work activity following the myocardial infarction. This nonreturn to work because of secondary gain can often be prevented by counseling prior to vocational decision making.

Programmatically, the assessment of the vocational ramifications for the coronary patient can be performed with a variety of tools. For example, assessment of the patient's job satisfaction, value of work, and job satisfactoriness provide a profile of contributing factors to a work return. Such factors can be measured by standardized assessments such as the Brayfield Job Satisfaction Scale and the Bowling Green Work Valuation Scale as well as nonstandardized tools such as employer interviews. Caution must be given regarding any standardized testing done in the coronary care process. Such assessments are significantly affected by emotional as well as environmental factors.

The patient's motivation to return to work may be determined by identifying the patient's perception of the utility or worth of a work return and the patient's perception of the probability of his returning to work successfully. Each of these factors should be assessed in relation to the patient's perception of the real or imagined economic, physical, or emotional costs created by the work return. This relationship can be characterized as shown on p. 142.

Motivational considerations

$$M = \frac{P(O_s) \times U}{C} = \text{Initiation of behavioral events; appraisal of rehabilitation concerns}$$

$P(O_s)$ = Probability of a successful outcome

U = Utility—usefulness, value, for example, work value—self-concept factors

C = Costs—psychological, physiological, and economical

Identification of these factors will not ensure a successful vocational decision, but it will increase the probability of knowing the patient better and of identifying potential secondary gains or covert fears of the patient. Likewise, a specific attempt to identify the relationship between job tasks and cardiopulmonary functioning should be made, using a systematic job analysis, within a reasonable amount of time (2 to 6 weeks following the myocardial infarction). The job analysis is the link between stress test findings, assessment of the coronary patient's emotional readiness to return to work, and the actual physical and psychological characteristics of the job. Such analysis should be done in two phases using a reliable format for gathering data. (See the boxed material.)

The first phase of the job analysis is performed with the patient. The interviewer reviews each question in detail to identify the patient's description of the physical as well as the psychological traits of the job. Special attention should be given to the patient's reaction to questions of job stress, method of returning to work, and work habits. The second phase of the job analysis should be performed at the patient's job site. This provides an objective view of the work site for the rehabilitation team. The patient may often subjectively embellish or reduce the work load characteristics in relation to the desire to return to work. The patient and employer must be active participants in the job analysis. The patient must also agree to have a member of the rehabilitation team visit the employer. It is also extremely desirable to make the job analysis a regular feature or cardiac rehabilitation programs, rather than just for "tough cases." The job analysis will dramatically illuminate vocational alternatives as well as methods to return to work for consideration by the patient during the adjustment process. The job analysis should be done prior to any stress test procedures and especially before any vocational decision making.

The fourth principle—*vocational rehabilitation services should be delivered by an interdisciplinary cardiac rehabilitation team*—acknowledges the complexity of the rehabilitation process as well as the different needs of patients. The rehabilitation of the coronary patient is a dynamic process of physical, social, emotional, and vocational adaptation. Each area, while being interactive, still requires a resource person to be available for consultation, as well as direct patient services. The rehabilitation team, consisting of the physician, coronary care nurse, physical therapist, occupational therapist, rehabilitation counselor, and

CARDIAC REHABILITATION OCCUPATIONAL STRESS INVENTORY

Patient's name ______________________ Case number ____________
Occupation ______________________ D.O.T. number __________
Stress-tested functional capacity ______________________
Functional therapeutic classification ______________________

1. Summary of duties ______________________

2. Actual tasks performed on job and job setup ______________________

3. Describe specific work area (e.g., temp-ventilation, clearance, traffic)

4. Describe surrounding work areas (e.g., entrance and exit areas—distance)

5. Machines, tools, instruments, devices used (e.g., wt., noise, power source, discharge) ______________________

6. Actual technique for task completion (e.g., upper, lower extremity use, rotation of trunk) ______________________

7. Energy requirements for job tasks (regular—emergency) (e.g., lifting, walking in Mets, KPM kilo/min) ______________________

8. What other types of job classes are involved in performance of job (e.g., aids, helpers, secretaries)? ______________________

9. What specific occupational groups can this job be broken into? __________

10. What jobs should lead to promotion to this job? ______________________

11. What lines of promotion are open on this job? ______________________

12. What are qualifications of job? ______________________

13. What occupation demands same type of training in other industries? ______

14. Hours of work/day ______________ /week ______________
    overtime requirements ______________________
15. Rate of pay ______________ union affiliation ______________
16. Supervised by ______________ lunch and break time ______________
17. Supervises ____________ (number of people)
    Apparent supervisory relationship ______________________

Continued.

CARDIAC REHABILITATION OCCUPATIONAL STRESS INVENTORY—cont'd

18. Vacation ______________________ shift schedule ______________
19. Method of travel to work ______________________
20. Rate of work required (e.g., piece rate/hr., work cycles, seasonal aspects)
____
21. Apparent psychological stress on job:

	None					Total
Role ambiguity	0	1	2	3	4	5
Under utilization	0	1	2	3	4	5
Overload	0	1	2	3	4	5
Resource inadequacy	0	1	2	3	4	5
Job insecurity	0	1	2	3	4	5
Nonparticipation	0	1	2	3	4	5
Reported job satisfaction	0	1	2	3	4	5
Reported value of work	0	1	2	3	4	5

22. Benefits available: Sick leave ______________________
Disability ______________________
Retirement ______________________
23. Company policy as to coronary cases ______________________
____
____
24. Does patient expect to return to work? ______________________
How ______________________
When ______________________
25. Specific recommendations for job modification or job return ______________
____
____

exercise physiologist, bridge the hospital/community transition. All too often, special hospital programs for the coronary patient do not offer the transitional as well as follow-up services needed for appropriate work return.

As a rehabilitation counselor, whether working for a state vocational rehabilitation agency or for a private rehabilitation agency, a professional rehabilitation specialist has an opportunity to significantly contribute to the vocational as well as personal adjustment of coronary patients. The counselor role within a cardiac rehabilitation team offers each of the other professions a window into the specificity of vocational planning following the coronary event. The use of a cardiac rehabilitation team contributes to the timely as well as the effective application of rehabilitation functions that will direct the patient toward health and well-being.

REFERENCES

1. Acker, J. E.: Factors affecting the employment of patients treated in coronary care units for myocardial infarction, J. Tenn. Med. Assoc. **61**:1200, 1968.
2. Adsett, A. C., and Bruhn, J. G.: Short-term group psychotherapy for postmyocardial infarction patients and their wives, Calif. Med. Assoc. J. **99**(12):577-584, 1968.
3. Aldes, J., Stein, S., and Grobin, S.: The rehabilitation of cardiac patients. Final Report, Project No. RD 1991-M, February, 1970.
4. Beck, A.: Cognitive therapy and the emotional disorders, New York, 1976, International Universities Press.
5. Cassem, N. H., and Hackett, T. P.: Psychiatric consultation in a coronary care unit, Ann. Intern. Med. **75**:9-14, 1971.
6. Cay, E. L., et al.: Return to work after a heart attack, J. Psychosom. Res. **17**:231, 1973.
7. Conley, R., and Nobel, J.: Workers' compensation reform challenge for the 80's, Am. Rehabil. **3**:19, 1978.
8. Croog, S., Levine, S., and Lurie, Z.: The heart patient and the recovery process, Soc. Sci. Med. **2**:111-164, 1968.
9. Croog, S., Shapiro, D., and Levine, S.: Denial among male heart patients, Psychosom. Med. **33**(5):385-397, 1971.
10. Garrity, T.: Vocational adjustment after first myocardial infarction; comparative assessment of several variables suggested in the literature, Soc. Sci. Med. **3**:705-717, 1973.
11. Gelfand, D., and Hagen, J.: Factors relating to unsuccessful vocational adjustment of cardiac patients, J. Occup. Med. **2**:62-70, 1960.
12. Hackett, T. P., and Cassem, N. H.: Psychological adaptation to convalescence in myocardial infarction patients. In Naughton, J., and Hellerstein, H., editors: Exercise testing and exercise training in coronary artery disease, New York, 1973, Academic Press Inc.
13. Havinghurst, T.: Human development and education, New York, 1953, David McKay, Inc.
14. Ibrahim, M., et al.: Management after myocardial infarction: a controlled trial of the effect of group psychotherapy, Int. J. Psychiatry Med. **5**(3):253-268, 1974.
15. Klein, R., and Dean, A.: The physician and post-myocardial infarction invalidism, J.A.M.A. **194**(2):123-128, 1966.
16. Kushner, B., et al.: The influence of psychological factors and early hospital follow-up on return to work after first myocardial infarction, Scand. J. Rehabil. Med. **7**(4):158-162, 1975.
17. Lazarus, A.: Behavior therapy and beyond, New York, 1971, McGraw-Hill Book Co.
18. Lazarus, A.: Multimodal behavior therapy: treating the B.A.S.I.C. I.D., J. Nerv. Ment. Dis. **156**:404-411, 1973.
19. Lazarus, A.: Multimodal behavior therapy, New York, 1976, Springer-Verlag New York, Inc.
20. Lazarus, A.: Personal comment, Multimodal Therapy Institute, Princeton, N.J., 1977.
21. Meichenbaum, D.: Cognitive behavior modification, New York, 1977, Plenum Publishing Corp.
22. Mitchell, K.: Motivational factors of a successful return to work after a myocardial infarction. Unpublished Doctoral Dissertation, Pennsylvania State University, 1975.
23. Mitchell, K.: Motivational factors in cardiac

rehabilitation, paper presented at American Congress of Rehabilitation Medicine, San Diego, 1976.
24. Mitchell, K.: Cardiac Rehabilitation: a multimodal approach, paper presented at American Congress of Rehabilitation Medicine, Miami, November, 1977.
25. Muir, J. R.: The rehabilitation of cardiac patients, Proc. R. Soc. Med. **70**(9):655-656, 1977.
26. Nagel, R., Gargola, R., and Picton-Robinson, I.: Factors influencing return to work after myocardial infarction, Lancet **2:**454, 1971.
27. Nieves, L.: Assertiveness training in the multimodal therapy framework, Multimodal Institute, New Brunswick, N.J., 1977, Rutgers University.
28. Shapiro, S., and Weinblatt, E.: Return to work after the first myocardial infarction. Arch. Environ. Health **24:**17-26, 1972.
29. Shiller and Baker: Returning to work after myocardial infarction, Med. J. Aust. **1:**859, 1976.
30. Stern, M. J., Pascale, L., and McLoone, J. B.: Psychosocial adaptation following an acute myocardial infarction, J. Chron. Dis. **29**(8): 513-526, 1976.
31. Suinn, R., and Weigel, E.: The innovative therapies: critical and creative contributions, New York, 1974, Harper & Row Publishers, Inc.
32. Weinblatt, E., and Shapiro, S.: Return to work and work status following first myocardial infarction, Am. J. Public Health **56**(2): 169-185, 1966.
33. Weinblatt, E., Shapiro, S., and Frank, C. W.: Prognosis of women with newly diagnosed heart disease, Am. J. Public Health **63**(7): 577-593, 1973.
34. Wenger, N. K., and Hellerstein, H. K.: Uncomplicated myocardial infarction, J. A.M.A. **224:**511-514, 1973.
35. Williamson, T. B.: The value of industrial rehabilitation following cardiac infarction, Proc. R. Soc. Med. **70**(9):656-657, 1977.
36. Wishnie, H., and Hackett, T. D.: Psychological hazards of convalescence following myocardial infarction, J.A.M.A. **215**(8):1292-1296, 1971.

SECTION FOUR

INTERVENTION

9

Psychological intervention in myocardial infarction

THOMAS P. HACKETT
NED H. CASSEM

Since most patients hospitalized for myocardial infarction are neither psychotic nor severely neurotic and therefore do not manifest the type of behavior typically associated with psychological intervention, it is extremely important for health care personnel to educate themselves regarding the possible advantages of psychological intervention for the coronary patient. It is important to learn when a request for consultation is appropriate, to make the request, and to prepare the patient for psychological intervention.

There are two major factors that hamper psychological consultation: (1) few patients in medical and surgical settings think to ask directly for such intervention and (2) the common belief that psychiatrists and psychologists treat only serious mental conditions. Most people believe that psychiatric assistance is required only when a problem gets out of hand. As a consequence, when an otherwise normal medical or surgical patient is seen by a psychiatrist because the general practitioner or internist has requested an evaluation, the patient is apt to be defensive and resistant because he sees the visit as a sign that his physicians have labeled him unstable. As yet psychiatrists have not made their mark as students or normal coping behavior. Their reputation and the specialty are identified with the psychotic or obviously disturbed patient. Psychiatrists are generally referred to patients by intermediaries such as physicians or nurses. Seldom does the patient himself see the need for psychological assistance. It therefore becomes extremely important that the patient be adequately prepared for a requested consultation. Whenever a physician or nurse wants a patient to be seen by a psychiatrist, the patient must be told why and must also be given an explanation of the role of the psychologist or psychiatrist in the coronary care unit. In

Prepared under Contracts PHS 43-67-1443 and HE 13781 of the National Institutes of Health, Public Health Service, United States Department of Health, Education and Welfare.

many intensive care settings in which psychiatric consultations are common, the routine nature of the visit can be stressed. The important point to be communicated is that a request for psychological intervention does not mean that the patient is in serious emotional difficulty. On the contrary, psychologists and psychiatrists have become more and more interested in assisting quite stable patients who are experiencing temporary difficulty in coping with a stressful event such as cardiac arrest or major surgery.

The best time for intervention is as soon as the patient begins to have trouble dealing with his medical or surgical problem—when he employs maladaptive coping patterns or when his means of coping fails to work. This is by no means as simple as it may sound. The signs of failure to cope are anxiety, depression, and regression—the common triad of reactions to any type of hospitalization. These signs of distress may not be obvious. Patients may hide them, may be unaware of their maladaptive behavior, or may be aware that something is wrong but be unable to ask for help. Many people are not tuned in to their psychological needs. Others are ashamed to admit to emotion or to display anxiety. Some dread being scorned because of their nervous condition. Often a cry for help takes the form of a distress signal that may be bizarre in nature. For example, some patients, failing to receive the kind of attention they want, try to sign out against medical advice.[1] Patients call attention to their emotional needs in many different ways. Some of these are determined by age, others by educational background, and still others by ethnic background. We have found, for example, that blue-collar workers are less apt to ask questions than are their white-collar counterparts.[7] It has been pointed out that the experience of pain is reported differently by members of different ethnic groups.[13] If this is true of pain, it is most likely true for emotional distress as well. In dealing with patients in distress it is most important to anticipate trouble and to intervene without being asked.

In describing the psychological problems of myocardial infarction, we have found it valuable to divide the experience into three phases. The first phase is the period prior to hospital admission and includes the time from the onset of symptoms to the patient's arrival at the doctor's office or the hospital. The second stage is the period of hospitalization. It is subdivided into the period in the emergency room, the period in the coronary care unit, and the period in the convalescent ward, including predischarge planning. The third phase is the convalescent phase, which extends from the moment of discharge to the return of maximum function at home, at work, and in the social world. Each of these phases presents its own problems and often its characteristic coping mechanisms. In our opinion, it is important to always keep in mind the specific phase in the experience. This awareness permits more accurate prediction of the problems more apt to occur at that point.

PREADMISSION

The principal problem posed in the preadmission phase is that of patient delay in seeking help. During the last 5 years a number of studies have explored this problem.[6,12,14] All findings agree that the average man or woman who experiences severe chest pain will delay 4 or 5 hours before seeking medical help. Since it is estimated that well over 60% of deaths caused by myocardial infarction occur from 30 to 60 minutes after the onset of chest pain, it is clear that delay of this sort is inappropriate as well as dangerous. It is estimated that at least 50% of these deaths could be prevented if patients were treated properly when the symptom develops.

As an example, consider the case of a couple in their sixties. The husband had suffered two previous heart attacks, and after each attack he had delayed seeking medical attention for hours. The symptoms of his third infarction began when he and his wife were hurrying to the Boston symphony on a Friday afternoon. The patient, a retired paper pulp mill executive, experienced severe precordial pain after the first block of exercise. By the time they reached the symphony hall, he was complaining of indigestion. His wife had heard that complaint once before and had failed to take action, even though she strongly suspected the problem was her husband's heart. The couple went into the performance, during which the patient sweated and squirmed. At the intermission, he blamed his condition on a hastily eaten lunch, but his wife continued to insist that it was his heart. She did not, however, call an attendant or an ambulance. On the way to the garage after the performance, the patient collapsed and was taken to a hospital, where he was successfully treated for his third myocardial infarction. Had his wife responded with more alacrity, she would have lessened the risk of her husband's dying before reaching the hospital.

Clinicians who have investigated the phenomenon of delay agree that the problem is entirely psychological. It is not caused by traffic, difficulty in locating a physician, or finding transportation. In our study and in others as well, the phenomenon of delay cuts across all the usual socioeconomic variables. Age, sex, level of education, socioeconomic status, and even history of a previous heart attack do not appear to reduce the tendency to delay. Most of the 4 or 5 hours are spent trying to decide whether or not to call a doctor. The decision-making process gets jammed by the patient's inability to admit that he is mortally sick.

Preadmission interventions

How can the patient be encouraged to seek medical treatment immediately? Everyone, and especially individuals in high-risk categories, must be taught to avoid looking for noncardiac explanations for chest pain. They must recognize this nonproductive search as denial when symptoms persist beyond 3 minutes.

They must learn to call a doctor without hesitation. Individual physicians must reassure their patients that this kind of call is always appropriate and is never an imposition.

An important further point is education of the entire population to aid in speeding coronary patients to a source of help. In our study[6] we found that of all the factors that work in favor of getting an individual to respond promptly, the most effective is the advice of another party. The more impersonal and authoritative that party is, the better. Policemen, foremen, nurses—all have better track records than do husbands or wives. In our study, wives seemed to have the least influence in persuading their husbands to call a physician. We therefore recommend that everyone, whether family or friend, take the initiative for the patient. We would encourage them to call an ambulance even before trying to persuade the patient that this course is imperative.

The all-important principle of intervention here is anticipation. If one can predict that the patient with chest pain will instantly perceive it as indigestion, it is then possible to alert him to the mortal danger of maintaining that rationalization for any longer than 3 to 5 minutes.

HOSPITALIZATION

Most individuals who arrive at a hospital with acute chest pain are immediately taken into an examining room where they are seen by a physician and cardiac monitoring is initiated. The instant care and concern demonstrated in the emergency room is most reassuring to coronary patients. The chief fear expressed by individuals in the emergency room is that of being left alone. Since this rarely happens, the emergency room experience is usually benign and swift. However, it is important to remember that if medical personnel must leave the room it is helpful to have an attendant or member of the family remain in the room with the patient.

Time spent in the coronary care unit is the second phase in the hospital experience, and it presents three principal sources of stress: (1) being monitored, (2) witnessing a cardiac arrest, and (3) experiencing a cardiac arrest. All can produce anxiety. Departure from the coronary care unit may also cause distress, a fact that has been substantiated by biochemical studies.[11] This is an important fact to remember because so often the patient regards transfer from the unit as a graduation, an indication that his heart is sufficiently steady and strong to be on its own. However, underlying this superficial happiness may be a profound concern for the lack of close monitoring and the reduced number of nurses on the convalescent ward to which he is assigned.

Psychiatrists are most commonly asked to assist patients whose anxiety or depression is obvious. As has been observed and expressed elsewhere, the symptom of anxiety is not usually evident in its virulent form in the coronary care unit.[9] While it may not be openly expressed, it is generally admitted to on questioning. Rarely does it take the form of tremulousness, fidgeting, hyperventilation, stammering, or sweating. It usually occurs on the first or the second day in the unit and its intensity declines thereafter, generally in conjunction with the rise of the defense of denial.[4] Denial is the repudiation of part or all of the available meaning of an event to reduce painful affect such as anxiety.[17] Denial can be conscious or unconscious. It may on the one hand be a complete lack of awareness of danger; on the other hand it may be manifested as a negation or deliberate minimization of the danger inherent in a given situation. An individual may have the ability to cast frightening thoughts from his mind and to concentrate on more pleasant things. He may, without being aware of making an effort to do so, simply not be aware of danger. Denial is commonly found among patients in the coronary care unit and accounts for their apparent serenity. The use of denial as a defense has been found to be a salutary influence. Its successful use correlates positively with increased rates of survival in the coronary care unit.[18] However, denial does not always come in a pure form. If it is successful, the individual will appear to be in no distress and will genuinely feel no distress. However, if it is not working well, the individual will admit to experiencing emotional distress during the course of an interview.

Depression ordinarily appears between the patient's fourth and fifth days in the coronary care unit, continues on through the sixth day, and may persist thereafter. It is important to note that periods of anxiety may also occur in response to various events in the unit or in the patient's life.

Together with anxiety and depression, problems of management, especially those caused by regression, are also frequent reasons for consultation. These problems usually appear after a patient has been in the unit for several days. Management problems center around three issues: signing out against advice, sexual misbehavior, and passive hostile-dependent problems. When a patient signs out against advice, he usually denies that his heart is as seriously damaged as the doctors claim. Sexual misbehavior generally takes the form of exhibitionism, suggestive language, and obscene remarks to the nurses. Management problems are more varied with patients who have passive hostile-dependent problems. Such patients are basically passive-aggressive individuals. Some are aggressive men who dislike being confined to bed and constantly test the limits imposed on the range of activity they are allowed.

Interventions for hospitalized patients

We have used a variety of psychological interventions in our work with hospitalized coronary patients. These can be divided into nine primary areas or methods of approach.

Education and explanation. This is the most common and perhaps the most important of all interventions. Much of the explaining has little to do with psychology but is done to reinforce survival essentials in the coronary care unit. For example, most patients are told within hours after entering the unit that loose electrodes can cause false alarms and that static on the monitor screen is more apt to stem from a misplaced electrode than from the heart. Nonetheless, we go over in detail the various pieces of equipment in the patient's immediate vicinity. We have found that the monitor is perceived very differently by patients from different socioeconomic backgrounds. The white-collar patient can frequently separate artifact from irregularities of rhythm. The blue-collar patient is apt to misinterpret all erratic movements on the monitor screen as indicative of a problem with his heart. Some individuals misinterpret the careful monitoring of vital signs and believe that because their pulse is checked every hour, they are in immediate danger of dying. Others believe that being awakened for readings of vital signs during the night means that they are most apt to die in their sleep and that the nurses are therefore reading vital signs to try to keep them awake. White-collar workers are more apt to have specific information about the process of infarction and about the process of repair. Blue-collar patients seem to know about infarction but have no concept of cardiac repair and therefore visualize their heart as having a permanent hole punched in it by the infarct. Using diagrams provided by the American Heart Association and diagrams that we have devised, it has been possible to illustrate graphically the destruction of cardiac tissue and the process of repair and scar formation and correct such misconceptions.

Enhancing confidence in equipment as well as personnel. In our first investigation of patients in the coronary care unit (1958), we regarded the electrodyne monitor pacemaker as a formidable instrument.[3] We believed it was bound to inspire considerable apprehension in the patients attached to it, and our prediction was that a high percentage of such patients would be anxious, would voice their anxiety, and would ask to have the machine removed. The results of a preliminary study did nothing to confirm our suspicions, and our findings were the opposite of our expectations. Far more patients were reassured by the monitor than frightened by it. Even those who underwent painful external pacing regarded the machine with a mixture of awe and gratitude. They did not view it as tangible evidence that their failing myocardium needed continual care and were frequently able to regard it as a mechanical guardian angel. The sick patient characteristically is able to fix on the benefit derived from a particular instrument and to negate its more threatening aspect, particularly if it causes no pain. The monitor is usually introduced as a benign mechanical support. The patient is told that the heart of every patient in the coronary care unit is continuously monitored and that the monitor acts as an ever-vigilant friend to alert the nurses to the slightest imperfection in rate or rhythm. The same type of explanation is given regarding other items of equipment. It has been our experience, and the experience of others as well, that the coronary care unit environment is more reassuring than fearful. It is our belief that the better the patient understands the purpose and function of the mechanical devices in the unit, the more able he will be to conquer fear. Very few patients object to the monitor, and visitors are more apt to be intimidated by the equipment than are patients.

Patients respond positively to coronary care unit personnel as well as to the equipment. They tend to view the physician and nurse as omnipotent. If this positive attitude is shaped by the psychological consultant, it can be converted into a realistically based powerful instrument for reassurance.

Confrontation. Confrontation is a technique that is commonly applied to problems of patient management. Men not infrequently feel "less than a man" after a myocardial infarction. To prove their masculinity they may flirt with nurses seductively, use four-letter words, tell gross jokes, and behave both in a provocative and sexually aggressive manner. Female nurses are advised to ask the patient if he realizes how sexually toned his language is or how often the subject of sex comes into his behavior. A nurse may tell the patient that even though she likes him as a person she does not like to be regarded as a sexual object. This confrontation is often enough to alter the individual's behavior. If it persists and the patient denies the problem, we have found it helpful to have a group confrontation in which the psychiatrist and a group of nurses talk with the patient together, beginning with the statement of their concern for the patient and their regard for him. This introduction is followed by observations about his comments and behavior. This technique has invariably been successful, even though individual patients do not always admit that their talk is as sexual as described.

Hypnosis. Hypnosis is all to infrequently used in the coronary care unit. Perhaps this is a reflection of its infrequent use in medicine in general. It is particularly helpful for the coronary patient because there are no medical side effects. We have used it to induce relaxation and to reduce anxiety. The general technique is to determine the hypnotizability of the subject by using the Spiegel eyeroll test and by doing rapid induction.[15] This process is preceded by an explanation of hypnosis and is never attempted without the full cooperation of the patient. If the patient is a good subject, he is taught autohypnosis. It is possible to use various objects in the unit as additional or ancillary sources for deepening the trance. For example, the beeper on the monitoring system can be incorporated into trance induction and become a pleasant sound.

Drugs. Although it is our observation that acute anxiety is fairly rare in coronary care unit patients, we advise routine sedation because mild to moderate anxiety is undoubtedly more common than the outward appearance of patients in the unit might suggest. Since it is unreasonable to expect the busy practitioner to spend enough time with each patient to unearth covert anxiety, we believe it is advisable to regard every patient as anxious and to treat him accordingly, even though supporting evidence might be lacking. It has been our custom to use a mild tranquilizer (diazepam, 5 mg 4 times daily, or chlordiazepoxide, 10 mg 4 times daily), which is to be administered on a regular basis with the stipulation that it can be deleted or decreased at the patient's request. Some patients dislike the feeling of being drugged and prefer some anxiety to drug-induced somnolence. Others equate drowsiness with weakness and think that drug-induced drowsiness is a sign that their heart is not operating effectively. For these few patients, tranquilization may not be the treatment of choice.

We have found the benzodiazepine group of tranquilizers to be the most effective because these drugs have fewer side effects than barbiturates and do not interfere with the effects of warfarin compounds. With their use, however, one must be alert to the possibility of a possible paradoxical effect, rage or a lowered threshold for anger.[16] This response has been rarely encountered in our experience. It is useful to remember that bedtime sedation can often be provided by doubling or tripling the sedative dose of the benzodiazepines. Flurazepam (Dalmane), because it exerts a minimal interference with REM sleep, has been widely used in intensive care settings and is considered a good hypnotic with a minimum number of side effects. In prescribing tranquilizers, we have found it necessary to emphasize the importance of mental rest in the coronary care unit and to assure patients that the administration of tranquilizers is part of the standard mode of treatment in the unit. There are some men who equate the need for sedation with a lack of manliness. This is an attitude that we do our best to dissipate. Antidepressants of the tricyclic group are contraindicated in the acute phase of coronary disease because their use has been linked with the occurrence of sudden death and arrhythmias. The same is true for the phenothiazines.

Exercise training. Passive range-of-motion exercises can be started in the coronary care unit on the first day following infarction in uncomplicated cases. A more active program can be developed thereafter, but as yet this is practiced in only a small number of hospitals. As activity becomes more accepted, which will occur in direct proportion to its safety, it will become more common. Activity in the coronary care unit has a number of values, the most important being that it allows the patient to feel that he is an active participant in his own program of recovery. He can see on a day-to-day basis that his disease does not proscribe physical activity.

Family therapy. Families often fear the hospital equipment in the coronary care unit more than the patients do. A brief discussion of the equipment with them would be time well spent. Before discharge, the spouse should be cautioned to avoid overprotecting or babying the patient. Families should also be told to expect a certain irritability on the part of the patient when his every need is not instantly attended to. Furthermore, a list of common misconceptions should be reviewed and corrected. Commonly held myths to be discredited are: (1) even mild exertion is dangerous and liable to cause sudden death; (2) driving must be avoided; (3) the arms must not be raised above the head, especially the left arm; (4) sexual intercourse should never again be attempted—if it is, repeat infarcts or sudden death tend to occur at orgasm; (5) recurrences are apt to occur on the anniversary of the first infarction; (6) the patient is liable to die at the same age as one of his parents or siblings; and (7) in sleep the heart is more vulnerable to recurrent infarction and sudden death. Time should be taken to question the patient and family about relatives or friends who have suffered an infarction to determine what their lives have been like in the wake of this disease. There is often a tendency for patient and family to identify with relatives or other victims and to foresee a similar outcome for themselves, even if the cases were quite dissimilar.

It is good to make sure that both the patient and the family realize what the possibilities are for the future to avoid discrepancies between the patient's estimate of his capacity and the family's thoughts on the matter. Such discrepancies do nothing but impair the rehabilitation process. When the patient and the family hear the instructions together, there is less likelihood that conflicts will occur. It is also wise to give couples specific information about sexual function and an adequate account of the pros and cons. They should be urged to return to an active sexual life if they have the inclination. In general, the more accurate instruction about all aspects of coronary disease, the better.

Support and respect for patients' personal needs. Generally coronary care unit patients receive a great deal of support from nurses and other personnel in the unit. Since the most quiet time of the diurnal-nocturnal cycle is in the late evening, we have made it a policy to telephone particularly distressed patients around 10 P.M. to check on their condition and let them know that we are thinking about them.

It is important, whenever possible, to provide each patient with the most pleasant possible daily routine—to provide art materials if he likes to draw, appropriate books if he likes to read, television, radio, and the like. Equally important is concern about his visitors. It is important to exclude people the patient does not want to see and to arrange screens at the door, if he has a private room, to keep people out. If the patient is in a four-bed ward, care must be taken to see that visitors to other patients are not too noisy or distressing.

In the case of certain businessmen who are used to being extremely active, who feel that their business is in jeopardy because of their hospitalization, and who clamor for a telephone, sometimes a telephone is installed in an effort to reduce their frustration. Similarly, we have allowed business conferences to be held in the coronary care unit as long as the patient's coronary condition remained stabilized.

Since the use of coronary artery bypass graft surgery, a sizable number of people who would formerly have been untreatable coronary invalids are now able to consider the possibility of regaining their previous activity level. This hope can be augmented by pointing out persons who have returned to an active work and social life. Presidents Eisenhower and Johnson can be included in this group. Both of these men illustrate the potential success of rehabilitation. There are also splendid examples of patients who have recovered from a myocardial infarction and later complete the Boston Marathon. This fact usually comes as a pleasant surprise to patients who enjoy athletics and fear a future of inactivity. The physician's interest in communicating the positive prognosis will do much to give a patient faith in his future rehabilitation.

Instruction in the art of antcipation. We have discussed the need for health care personnel to anticipate the emotional problems of their patients. It is of paramount importance for the patient to also be taught the art of anticipation. If a possible problem is foreseen, it can be met with some equanimity—the sting has been removed. Anticipation can be a valuable ally in the rite of passage through emergency room, coronary care unit, convalescent ward, and back home.

CONVALESCENCE

The chief bugbear of convalescence from a psychiatric point of view is depression. Paul Dudley White has said, "It is of importance to realize that the heart may recover more rapidly than the depressed mental state which is so often a complication."[18] The depressed state of mind is a major concern in the psychological rehabilitation of patients who have suffered an acute myocardial infarction. We share the conviction of Hellerstein that feelings of depression are "virtually universal in the period following onset of infarction."[10] It becomes particularly obvious when the patient leaves the hospital and returns home.

The depression that occurs in the wake of a myocardial infarction is reactive and exogenous in type. Like grief following the loss of a loved one, this depression is an appropriate response. It is most certainly not abnormal or neurotic to be depressed after a coronary attack. It is clearly distinct from endogenous depressive reactions; these are apt to be cyclical and unpredictable in origin and require different management.

The principal danger in all depressions is suicide. Although there are not studies that cite the incidence of suicide in patients subsequent to myocardial infarction, it is our opinion that deliberate self-destructive acts are unusual in this population. Rather, the course of the depression, if plotted on a graph, would resemble a plateau with few ups and downs and a gradual slope returning to a baseline of normal in from 3 to 6 months.

The basis for postinfarction depression is, in our opinion, the threat of invalidism and the loss of autonomy and independence. The sooner the patient's sense of self-esteem is restored, the more rapidly the depression will resolve.

There is no better approach to this task than to make the patient active again.

The patient is involved in very little activity in the hospital. Aside from walking the length of the ward at irregular intervals during the convalescent stage, the patient is encouraged to remain recumbent and to relax most of the time. As a consequence, when the patient is discharged from the hospital he is in poor physiological condition to begin a program of much exercise. He develops what we have termed the homecoming depression, the principal symptom of which is weakness.[20] The feeling of weakness itself is described as one of exhaustion or physical weakness with minimal effort. It is often regarded by patients as a harbinger of cardiac decline, and this sense of weakness is often the trigger that shoots an underlying depression into the open. The symptom of weakness must stem from a variety of sources. Deranged cardiovascular physiology resulting from the myocardial infarction must play a part, as must the inactivity typical of coronary convalescence. Since a feeling of weakness is a cardinal symptom of depression, it is probable that this also adds to the pervasive sense of exhaustion. Easy fatigue also accentuates the patient's underlying fear that he might soon become a cardiac cripple.

The prospect of reduced physical activity would pose no concern to the laggard, the dawdler, or the leisure-seeker. However, we know of no study that describes the coronary patient as indolent, listless, or lazy. Most research, especially the work of Friedman and Rosenman,[5] points to the exact opposite traits as common to coronary-prone people. They are work addicts with a keen awareness of time and deadline. They are seldom able to relax, even on vacation. For this reason, a restriction of either physical or mental activity imposes an enormous tax on their emotional economy.

There are other sources of stress that are characteristic of the immediate convalescent phase. These are (1) the threat of sudden death, (2) depression caused by job uncertainty, sexual insecurity, and family role reversal (for example, the wife frequently must provide the family's sole financial support), and (3) depressions caused by deprivations (cigarettes, food, and excitement). Add these to the homecoming depression, and the patient's burden is such that he is almost forced to view himself as a cardiac cripple—a damaged man.

Convalescence interventions

Our goals in therapy or the goals of intervention are to restore self-confidence and to reinstate a positive self-image through the use of physical conditioning.

Exercise programs and physical conditioning. Exercise and physical conditioning are perhaps the most crucial interventions in helping the patient to attain a renewed feeling of independence and rehabilitative progress. They are the prime adversary of depression. One of the most important features of physical conditioning is that it precludes empty days in convalescence. A skilled nurse or physical therapist can be most specific in setting up a regimen to satisfy the compulsive patient. Physical activity can provide a welcome "do" in the long list of "don'ts" (don't smoke, don't eat too much, don't hurry, don't worry). In the final analysis, living is moving, and depression stands against life and motion.

Medication. Most patients are sent home from the hospital without the assistance of either a tranquilizer to help them deal with homecoming stress or a hypnotic to guarantee sound sleep. This seems a singular oversight, since physicians are well aware of the regularity with which sleep disturbances plague the patient recovering from infarction during his first few months at home. We are convinced of the importance of prescribing these medications and of encouraging patients to make good use of them. The benzodiazepines, when used correctly, are nonaddicting and are a good antidote to emotional stress and its resulting irritability. The phenothiazines are to be avoided, however, since they possess hypotensive properties and increase cardiac irritability.

In the treatment of depression in the coronary patient, it is wise to avoid the tricyclic antidepressants since it seems fairly clear that they can be associated with arrhythmias and sudden death.[19] It has been said that doxepin has been free of association with such cardiac side effects, but this has not as yet been carefully documented. It is therefore important to consider other means of combating depression. It is possible that diazepam and chlordiazepoxide can be effective in the treatment of depression as well as in the treatment of anxiety, but this has not proved true for all patients by any means. If used, they should most certainly be supported by additional forms of therapy.

Follow-up telephone calls to patient and family. Telephone calls are made every week for the first month or two following discharge. Usually a nurse-clinician who has met the patient and his family during his hospitalization phones at a designated time. She talks with both patient and spouse to ask specific questions. Many issues arise about which the patient would not ordinarily feel justified in bothering the doctor. Nonetheless these problems need answers. The patient wonders how far he can safely proceed with his physical conditioning program. He is unclear about the advisability of sexual activity. He wants to know about walking his dog (there is a difference between walking a Great Dane and a Chihuahua). He wants to know what his doctor meant by "take it easy." It is also wise to set aside a specific time when the patient or his spouse can feel free to call the nurse-clinician or the doctor.

Heart clubs. One possible resource that can assist the patient in counteracting depression and in restoring a sense of well-being and self-esteem are "heart clubs."[2] Such groups are weekly forums in which eight or ten patients with similar problems can exchange information under the supervision of a nurse-clinician as they learn to live with their cardiac problem.

Reinforcement of intervention begun in the hospital. It is important to remind the patient of the 47 members of the United States Senate who have suffered heart attacks and of celebrities such as Peter Sellers and Pearl Bailey whose recovery and return to active schedules can be cited. The patient should be helped to see that he is most certainly not alone. Continued support and expression of interest is crucial.

The continued use of relaxation techniques learned in the hospital should be encouraged. These techniques, whether they be transcendental meditation, self-hypnosis, or simply a nap in the middle of the day, are quite valuable. It is good to suggest that the patient set aside a time each day to relax and to think about what he is doing, to consciously avoid stress, and to continue to work to reduce the stress in his day. Continuing education about cardiac rehabilitation is also important. The patient can be referred to books on coronary disease, and liberal use should be made of the various pamphlets published by the American Heart Association. The all-important art of anticipation must once again be underlined. If the patient is told to expect a feeling of weakness on returning home from the hospital and that this is a normal response, much anguish can be spared.

REFERENCES

1. Albert, H. D., and Kornfeld, D. S.: The threat to sign out against medical advice, Ann. Intern. Med. **79:**888, 1973.
2. Bilodeau, C. B., and Hackett, T. P.: Issues raised in a group setting by patients recovering from myocardial infarction, Am. J. Psychiatry **128:**73, 1971.
3. Browne, I. W., and Hackett, T. P.: Emotional reactions to the threat of impending death: a study of patients on the monitor cardiac pacemaker, Irish J. Med. Sci. **496:**177, 1967.
4. Cassem, N. H., and Hackett, T. P.: Psychiatric consultation in a coronary care unit, Ann. Intern. Med. **75:**9, 1971.
5. Friedman, M.: Pathogenesis of coronary artery disease, New York, 1969, McGraw-Hill Book Co.
6. Hackett, T. P., and Cassem, N. H.: Factors contributing to delay in responding to signs and symptoms of acute myocardial infarction, Am. J. Cardiol. **24:**651, 1969.
7. Hackett, T. P., and Cassem, N. H.: White vs. blue collar responses to having a heart attack, Psychosom. Med. **34:**475, 1972.
8. Hackett, T. P., Cassem, N. H., and Wishnie, H. A.: The coronary care unit: an appraisal of its psychologic hazards, N. Engl. J. Med. **279:**1365, 1968.
9. Hackett, T. P., Cassem, N. H., and Wishnie, H. A.: Detection and treatment of anxiety in the coronary care unit, Am. Heart J. **78:**727, 1969.
10. Hellerstein, H. K.: Rehabilitation of the postinfarction patient, Hosp. Pract. **7:**45, 1972.
11. Klein, R. F., et al.: Transfer from a coronary care unit: some adverse responses, Arch. Intern. Med. **122:**104, 1968.
12. Moss, A. J., et al.: Delay in hospitalization during the acute coronary, Am. J. Cardiol. **24:**659, 1969.
13. Sborowski, M.: People in pain, San Francisco, 1969, Jossey-Bass Inc., Publishers.
14. Simon, A. B., et al.: Components of delay in the pre-hospital setting of acute myocardial infarction, Am. J. Cardiol. **30:**475, 1972.
15. Spiegel, H.: An eye-roll test for hypnotizability, Am. J. Clin. Hypn. **5:**25, 1972.
16. Tobin, J. M., et al.: Preliminary evaluation of librium in the treatment of anxiety reactions, Dis. Nerv. Syst. **21**(suppl. 2):11, 1960.
17. Weisman, A. D., and Hackett, T. P.: The predilection to death: death and dying as a psychiatric problem, Psychosom. Med. **23:**232, 1961.
18. White, P. D.: Heart disease, New York, 1951, Macmillan Inc.
19. Williams, R. B., and Sherter, C.: Cardiac complications of tricyclic antidepressant therapy, Ann. Intern. Med. **74:**395, 1971.
20. Wishnie, H. A., Hackett, T. P., and Cassem, N. H.: Psychological hazards of convalescence following myocardial infarction, J.A.M.A. **215:**1292, 1971.

10

Sexual counseling of coronary patients

CYNTHIA C. SCALZI
KATHLEEN DRACUP

The sexual act of intercourse is a natural biological function of life that provides a sense of intimacy and tender reassurance. The expressions of human sexuality—touching, holding, intercourse, fantasy—provide men and women with a weapon against feelings of isolation and worthlessness and offer a special place free of tension and stress. For patients with coronary disease, however, the exact opposite is often the case. Sexual intimacy, particularly coitus, is frequently seen as stressful and even life threatening. The fears and misconceptions harbored by coronary patients and their spouses, coupled with inadequate sexual counseling by physicians and nurses, serve to make sexual dysfunction following myocardial infarction a frequently noted phenomenon.

This chapter will describe the common sexual disorders seen in coronary patients, their causes, and the role of nursing and medical personnel in the prevention and treatment of such problems. Major emphasis will be placed on the need for and the process of sexual counseling. A framework for assessment of sexual difficulties and guidelines for patient instruction are provided. Also discussed will be the use of sexual therapy in the treatment of patients with prolonged sexual disorders such as impotence and inorgasmia.

SEXUAL DYSFUNCTIONS

Some of the sexual problems reported by coronary patients have been well documented in the medical literature.[1,5,14,16] The following discussion is not intended to cover all sexual disorders, only those most commonly experienced following a myocardial infarction.

Male disorders

The two major manifestations of sexual dysfunction in postcoronary men are erectile failure and premature ejaculation. Erectile difficulty may be experienced in varying degrees, including failure of the penis to harden sufficiently, loss of firmness after hardening, or complete flaccidity.[6,16] For the purposes of this discussion, we are referring to coronary patients with secondary impotence, that is, patients who functioned well before experiencing coronary disease. Premature ejaculation is cited in the literature as the most common of the male sexual dysfunctions.[6] Kaplan defines it as a condition wherein a man is unable to exert voluntary control over his ejaculatory reflex such that once he is sexually aroused, he reaches orgasm very quickly. Masters and Johnson[8] define a premature ejaculator as one who cannot control his ejaculatory process for a sufficient length of time to satisfy his partner in at least 50% of their coital experiences. Although reliable data supporting this disorder in a coronary population are not yet available, clinical experience suggests that secondary premature ejaculation is indeed quite prevalent in these patients.

Female disorders

Secondary inorgasmia is defined as an inability to achieve orgasm in situations in which similar arousal would have produced orgasm in the past. Again, despite the lack of documentation, clinical experience indicates that temporary secondary inorgasmia is frequently experienced by postcoronary females.

Decreased sexual desire

Decreased sexual desire is characterized by an inhibition of the general arousal aspect of the sexual response and is a commonly experienced phenomenon among both male and female postcoronary patients.[1,5,14,16] Both males and females experience impairment of the vasocongestive component of the sexual response. The female has difficulty lubricating, while the male experiences erectile difficulty.

The extent of sexual dysfunction in postcoronary patients is illustrated by two studies of male patients suffering myocardial infarction.[7,16] In the first study, of 20 patients studied from 3 months to 5 years after suffering an infarction, only five reported full resumption of sexual activity, seven claimed complete abstinence, and eight others reported a diminished level of intercourse. In the second study, 65% complained of a marked and lasting decline in sexual activity and 10% became permanently impotent.

FACTORS CONTRIBUTING TO SEXUAL DYSFUNCTION

Three factors can be easily identified in the development of secondary sexual problems in the postcoronary patient: (1) the patient's psychological response to coronary disease and the coronary event per se, (2) the physical limitations experienced by the individual as a result of the coronary episode, surgical intervention, and/or medication, and (3) the lack of information that contributes to fears and misconceptions about sexual functioning for the patient and the patient's spouse.

Psychological response

A number of psychosocial variables influence the coronary patient's sense of sexual health. After cardiac illness, the individual's sense of self-esteem and previously satisfying sexual relationship(s) may falter. The patient may fear imminent death and, in the face of this preoccupation, little mental or physical energy is left to deal with matters of sexuality. In group therapy sessions, convalescent male coronary patients have expressed feelings of diminished libido and fear of death during intercourse. They also frequently express feelings of anxiety that exist at a preconscious level for many years following their myocardial infarction, a feeling shared by their spouses.[1,3]

Almost all coronary patients who have suffered a myocardial infarction or undergone coronary revascularization experience depression during intensive care and immediately after hospitalization. This emotional state involves an inability to invest emotionally in another person(s), as well as feelings of guilt. Moreover, these feelings are further compounded by the forced dependency of the hospital setting and the oversolicitous spouse. The result is an erosion of feelings of self-worth and sexual attractiveness, for example, feelings that "I'm less of a man!" or "I'm not as feminine as I used to be." Nurses are familiar with the behavioral manifestations of such feelings when patients in the hospital setting repeatedly ask for recognition and approval of their maleness or femaleness.

In a study conducted by Hellerstein and Friedman,[5] 24 of 48 men who had suffered a myocardial infarction reported a significant decrease in the frequency of sexual activity. These individuals listed causes for this decline in sexual function that primarily related to their mental status following their attack: changes in their sexual desire, fear of having another coronary attack, feelings of depression, and fear on the part of their spouses. The importance of the spouse must not be ignored. Many husbands and wives of postcoronary patients find themselves in a psychologically traumatic situation, wanting to reassure their spouses of their love and concern, yet fearing the consequences of sexual activity. Their fears may be displaced into avoidance of sex, overprotection, or resentment of their responsibility for the health status of their partner. All of these factors combine to create a climate that may be more detrimental to the patient than the underlying cardiovascular pathology.

Physical limitations

The physical status of the postcoronary patient is the second factor that contributes to problems in successful resumption of sexual activity. Following myocardial infarction or vascular surgery, an individual often experiences extreme fatigue and weakness. If this fatigue is further complicated by cardiovascular symptoms such as chest pain (angina) on exertion and/or shortness of breath, the patient may fear the potential cost of sexual intercourse.

The question that must be answered in evaluating the patient's ability to safely resume sexual function is: What is the physiological cost of intercourse? The first significant experimental findings describing the impact of sexual activity on physiological status were reported by Hellerstein and Friedman.[5] They studied 48 postcoronary patients and 43 normal, coronary-prone individuals to determine the differential effects of sexual versus other daily activities on human physiology. Among their conclusions was the fact that in both groups the cost of sexual intercourse was quite modest for these middle-aged, middle-class males married for many years. In the 14 patients monitored by Holter recording at home during coitus, heart rate response was minimal, with the peak rate averaging 117.4 beats per minute (range of 90 to 144 bpm). The average heart rate for the 2 minutes before orgasm and the 2 minutes after orgasm was 97.5 bpm (range of 85 to 102.2 bpm).

Blood pressure was measured during bicycle ergometry exercise tests at the heart rate recorded during intercourse. The average blood pressure level was 127/85 mm Hg at rest and 162/89 mm Hg at the peak heart rate for coitus. However, physical exercise such as riding a bicycle elevates the cuff blood pressure in the arms, but not the central aortic pressure.[11] Since this latter pressure can be elevated in sexual activity, the blood pressure findings reported here may not accurately reflect the situation during intercourse.

The oxygen uptake (in terms of percent of maximal oxygen consumption determined by bicycle ergometry) was 60.3% (16.0 ml of O_2 per kg) for the maximal heart rate and 45.3% (11.9 ml of O_2 per kg) for the average heart rate.

The average man who has recovered from an uncomplicated myocardial infarction has a maximum capacity of 8 to 9 Mets. The maximum heart rate activity during coitus is approximately 5 Mets for less than 30 seconds. During the preorgasm and postorgasm phases, the energy cost is only about 3.7 Mets. Thus, the energy expenditure associated with sexual activity for the typical postcoronary patient is relatively benign. If the coronary patient can walk on a treadmill at 3 to 4 miles per hour, climb stairs, or pass a Master's test without undue increase in blood pressure, heart rate, electrocardiogram changes, his exercise capacity is 5 to 6 Mets. This level of ability is well above the work requirements for sexual function.[4]

The individual's fatigue and experience of cardiovascular symptoms such as tachycardia during intercourse must be evaluated in light of the Hellerstein and Friedman findings.[5] The physician may want to prescribe nitroglycerin or propranolol to decrease the work load on the heart during sexual activity, rather than counsel abstinence. The medical and nursing personnel may also want to suggest a cardiac rehabilitation program involving specific exercise training. Research has shown that the physically conditioned postcoronary patient can perform a given level of work (including sexual intercourse) at a much lower heart rate and lower systolic blood pressure than is true of an untrained coronary patient.[15]

Lack of information

The third factor contributing to the wide occurrence of sexual dysfunction in postcoronary patients is inadequate sexual counseling by medical and nursing personnel. Health care professionals are for the most part still largely unaware of the enormous impact that physical illness may have on social and sexual functioning. The attitude that ill persons are not sexual plays a major role in the perpetuation of this nescience. Physicians and nurses working with coronary patients may inadvertently contribute to the patient's sexual difficulties by neglecting to discuss openly the impact of the disease on such activities. During the course of hospital convalescence the coronary patient begins to question his ability to return to normal daily functioning, including return to work, ability to undergo emotional stress, and capacity to perform physical activities involved in recreational pursuits and sexual intercourse. Without adequate sexual counseling, both the patient and the spouse must rely on their own (often limited) knowledge, myths, and misconceptions to cope with the uncertainty and fear of sexual inadequacy, impotence, and death during sexual intercourse.

In a study by Tuttle et al.[16] two thirds of the postcoronary patients interviewed received no advice whatsoever regarding sexual matters; the remaining one third received only vague and nonspecific advice. As illustrated by this study, many physicians and nurses give general advice such as "Take it easy!" and "Don't overdo when it comes to sex!", thereby shifting the ultimate decision about when and how to resume sexual activity to the patient.

The topic of human sexuality has traditionally been excluded from medical and nursing curricula. Many physicians and nurses have not been prepared, nor do they feel comfortable in assessing areas of sexual dysfunction and/or providing patients with specific information about sexual activity. By avoiding the issue or by giving vague advice, however, the health care team reinforces the patient's fears and anxieties. This approach leads to decreased sexual activity or problems in sexual function on the part of the patient, which in the main is physiologically unwarranted and psychologically detrimental.

The remainder of the chapter will focus on sexual counseling and its importance in preventing the development of secondary sexual disorders.

SEXUAL COUNSELING

The goal of sexual counseling is to provide the patient with the information he needs to *make his own choice* regarding sexual activity. The role of the medical staff and nurses is not to lay down rules concerning such activity, but rather to help the patient with his concerns (fears, anxieties, guilt) and lack of knowledge in this area.

Sexual counseling should be initiated early in the patient's hospitalization. The topic can be introduced soon after admission to the coronary care unit by informing the patient that most individuals who have suffered a coronary attack are able to return to usual or modified activities after a period of convalescence. Sexual activity is included in the list of such activities, along with work and social/recreational endeavors. Specifically, the topic of sexual activity should be included in the more general discussion of resumption of *physical* activities. If printed material, audio tapes, or other aides are used in conjunction with teaching about cardiac rehabilitation, it is helpful to also have a section under physical activity devoted to sexual function. Early inclusion of this subject matter may assist patients in verbalizing their questions, fears, and fantasies regarding future functioning (and perhaps dysfunctioning) in this area of interpersonal relationships and biological function. It also clearly identifies sexual activity as an area that will be discussed by medical and nursing personnel prior to discharge.

Separate counseling sessions for the coronary patient and the spouse are advantageous. Interviewing the couple individually provides the opportunity to express personal concerns that they may not feel comfortable sharing in the presence of their mate. Patients may be concerned about future extramarital or casual sexual experiences but are hesitant to discuss this in front of their spouse. Spouses, on the other hand, may be experiencing guilt if the coronary attack occurred during sexual intercourse or may be fearful of death during sexual intercourse on resumption of sexual activities, but do not want to burden their mate with such anxieties.

A joint counseling session prior to discharge assures the couple of hearing the same information and also gives the counselor the opportunity to reinforce advice given in the individual sessions.

Three sessions, therefore, for the purpose of sexual counseling are ideal. Some couples may not need all three, and counselors must be sensitive to the cues the couple gives in this regard. There is no standard that must be rigidly followed. Obviously, privacy is an essential component of counseling sessions, although this is often difficult to achieve in the usual hospital (especially the CCU) setting.

Assessment and instructions

Table 9 gives the general areas of assessment that we have found essential in sexual counseling. The rationale for the different assessment questions is presented along with guidelines for patient instruction.

In instructing coronary patients about resumption of sexual activity, as with

Table 9. Areas of assessment for sexual dysfunction in postcoronary patients*

Assessment	Rationale	Instructions
Previous patterns of sexual activity Availability of partner Frequency (times per week/month) Average duration (minutes) Usual time of day (AM/PM) Favored position(s)—MOT, MOB, side-to-side	Goal of counseling: return to precoronary level of sexual activity. Specific assessment of patterns gives baseline information that Indicates need for sexual counseling Identifies *previous* stressful sexual patterns Provides information needed to individualize instructions	General principle: intercourse like any other physical activity places a demand on cardiovascular system. Recommendations: Positions that impose less strain because of familiarity Avoid intercourse After a heavy meal After excessive alcohol intake When extremely fatigued Under time pressure With unfamiliar sexual partners†
Past experience with chest pain during sexual stimulation and/or intercourse	Not an uncommon experience if the patient has had chest pain during sexual activity; increased fear and anxiety may be anticipated in the patient and the partner	Instructions regarding the prophylactic use of nitroglycerin: Take prior to sexual intercourse or any activity that the patient knows might precipitate chest pain Information regarding the purpose, side effects, and how to take nitroglycerin
History of sexual difficulty 1-3 months prior to the heart attack Kind: women—inorgasmia; men—erectile difficulty, premature ejaculation Frequency: how many times in past 3 months Surrounding circumstances (stressful patterns) Medications—preinfarction and postinfarction Preexisting disease states that may cause sexual dysfunction, for example, diabetes	Previous sexual difficulty, particularly impotence in men, appears to be a common experience. Periodic, sporadic episodes of sexual difficulty are normal and commonly associated with fatigue and emotional stress. However, sexual difficulty prior to the infarction tends to increase fears of sexual inadequacy and permanent impotence. Some drugs that affect sexual response are: Reserpine: decrease libido and/or cause impotence Methyldopa: impotence, lack of sexual desire, and disorders of ejaculation Propranolol: increased fatigue with decreased sexual desire	Information should emphasize that this is a common experience that is frequently associated with stressful life patterns (fatigue, working long hours, emotional stress); under similar circumstances, this may occur periodically after a heart attack, particularly if there is anxiety

*From Scalzi, C., and Dracup, K.: Heart Lung 7(5):843, 1978.

†There is a greater physical and emotional stress caused by performance anxiety associated with new sexual experiences.

Table 9. Areas of assessment for sexual dysfunction in postcoronary patients—cont'd

Assessment	Rationale	Instructions
Patient's and partner's understanding of when they can resume sexual activity	To identify the expectations, information acquired, and misconceptions that may need to be clarified in the instructions	Resumption of sexual activity (6-8 weeks postinfarction‡ Physical conditioning programs enhance exercise tolerance and ability to participate in intercourse Warning signals patient should know and report to physician Rapid heart rate and/or rapid breathing that persists (4-5 minutes after orgasm) Feeling of extreme fatigue the day after intercourse Chest pain during or after intercourse

‡Also determined by the physician's assessment of the extent of recovery and the patient's ability to tolerate progression of physical activity.

other areas of cardiac rehabilitation, a multidisciplinary approach and follow-up of the patient and spouse are essential. Discharge often activates fears and concerns not experienced during hospitalization, and effective sexual counseling then occurs in the outpatient setting. This means that nurses working in expanded roles in community settings must be knowledgeable about such matters, both the issues of evaluation and the techniques of sexual counseling.

During the hospital and/or outpatient counseling sessions, medical or nursing personnel may diagnose the presence of long-standing and severe sexual dysfunction(s) about which he or she feels professionally unprepared to counsel the patient. A referral for appropriate sexual therapy can then be made if the patient or couple desires. It is important, however, to differentiate sexual counseling from sexual therapy, since physicians and nurses can have skills in the former without being expected to be "sex therapists."

To date, there have been no published studies supporting the therapeutic effectiveness of sexual counseling in postcoronary patients. However, an ongoing research program[12] suggests that patients who receive sexual counseling resume their precoronary level of sexual activity much quicker than do patients not exposed to this intervention. Clearly, more research needs to be done in this area of rehabilitation.

SEXUAL THERAPY

Sexual therapy has flourished in the past decade, stimulated by basic research[8,9] and a social climate in which public attention has focused on human sexuality. The brief, behaviorally oriented approaches to the treatment of sexual dysfunction[2,6] are based on the concept that such problems are caused by sexual ignorance, performance anxiety, and culturally influenced inhibition. It is widely accepted that sexual dysfunctions are more frequently caused by psychogenic problems than by physical illnesses. This knowledge has resulted in a justifiable enthusiasm for treating the *psychogenic* sexual disorders.

Until very recently, patients experiencing sexual dysfunction who were physically ill and disabled have been virtually ignored. However, increasing attention and clinical application of sexual therapy to patients with somatic problems suggest the potential for positive outcomes.[14]

One of the limitations of sexual therapy is that, in most university-based clinics, treatment entails the participation of two cooperative individuals. The prescribed exercises that are crucial elements of sexual therapy are essentially structured interactions between sex partners. They simply cannot be conducted alone. This often, therefore, poses a problem for the single (unmarried, separated, widowed) patient with a sexual disorder.

Since the educational and clinical requirements for training sexual therapists is from 1 to 2 years in most university-based programs, sexual therapy is understandably not a skill in the repertoire of most medical and nursing personnel. Nevertheless, it is realistic to expect physicians and nurses working with coronary patients (as well as other types of physically ill persons) to be able to assess sexual dysfunction in their patients and refer such persons to appropriate therapy centers. Such clinics are presently available in most large university medical centers across the United States and at present they provide the most reliable treatment for patients with sexual difficulties.

SUMMARY

The preceding discussion of sexual counseling with postcoronary patients emphasized the extent and nature of sexual disorders among male and female patients suffering from myocardial infarction and cardiovascular surgery. It also pointed out the three main causes of such disorders: psychological reactions of the patient, physiological limitations, and lack of factual information regarding sexual matters. The importance of adequate sexual counseling for both patients and their spouses was stressed, along with specific instructions for evaluation and counseling of various disorders (inorgasmia, premature ejaculation, impotence). The goal of sexual counseling is to help the patient and spouse make their own choices regarding the resumption of satisfying sexual relations. Counseling should be initiated early in the hospitalization and introduced within the context of a more general discussion about resumption of physical activities after coronary illness. Individual and joint counseling sessions are recommended, as well as outpatient follow-up. The differences between sexual counseling and sexual therapy were also pointed out.

REFERENCES

1. Adsett, C. A., and Bruhn, J. G.: Short-term psychotherapy for myocardial infarction patients and their wives, Can. Med. Assoc. J. **99:**577, 1968.
2. Annon, J. S.: The behavioral treatment of sexual problems: brief therapy, vol. 1, Honolulu, 1975, Enabling Systems, Inc.
3. Bilodeau, C. J., and Hackett, T. P.: Issues raised in a group setting by patients recovering from initial myocardial infarction, Am. J. Psychiatry **128:**73, 1971.
4. Green, A. W.: Sexual activity and the post-myocardial infarction patient, Am. Heart J. **89:**248, 1974.
5. Hellerstein, H. K., and Friedman, E. H.: Sexual activity and the postcoronary patient, Arch. Intern. Med. **125:**992, 1970.
6. Kaplan, H. S.: The new sex therapy, New York, 1974, Brunner-Mazel, Inc.
7. Klein, R. F., et al.:The physician and post-myocardial infarction invalidism, J.A.M.A. **194:**123, 1965.
8. Masters, W. H., and Johnson, V.: Human sexual inadequacy, Boston, 1970, Little, Brown & Co.
9. Masters, W. H., and Johnson, V.: Human sexual response, Boston, 1966, Little, Brown & Co.
10. Nemac, E., Mansfield, L., and Kennedy, J. W.: Heart rate and blood pressure responses during sexual activity in normal males, Am. Heart J. **92:**276, 1976.
11. Rowell, L. B., et al.: Disparities between aortic and peripheral pulse pressures included by upright exercise and vasomotor changes in man, Circulation **37:**954, 1968.
12. Scalzi, C.: Education and modification of risk behaviors in patients with ischemic heart disease, Grant No. 061774. Funded by American Heart Association, Greater Los Angeles Affiliate. Report in preparation.
13. Scalzi, C., and Dracup, K.: Sexual counseling of cardiac patients, Heart Lung. In press.
14. Scalzi, C., Loya, F., and Golden, J.: Sexual therapy of patients with cardiovascular disease, West. J. Med. **126:**243, 1977.
15. Stein, R. A.: The effect of exercise training on heart rate during coitus in the post-myocardial infarction patient, Circulation **55:** 738, 1977.
16. Tuttle, W. B., Cook, W. L., and Fitch, E.: Sexual behavior in postmyocardial infarction patients, Am. J. Cardiol. **13:**140, 1964.

11

Behavioral approaches to risk reduction in coronary patients

CAROLE SCHORNAGEL ORLEANS

Findings of epidemiological and experimental studies published over the past decade, too numerous and complex to review here, have implicated a number of *behavioral* risk factors in cardiovascular disease.[2,4] Two classes of preventable risk factors have been established:[51] (1) risk factors related to life-style and culturally sanctioned habits including cigarette smoking; diet excessive in calories, saturated fat, and cholesterol intake; sedentary life-style; and the type A behavior pattern characterized by impatience, excessive job involvement, and a hard-driving, competitive attitude and (2) risk factors related to impaired biochemical-physiological processes such as hypertension, hyperlipidemia, and diabetes that are potentially amenable to external influences such as diet, medication, and altering of life-style. Synthesizing the research findings concerning these two classes of risk factors, investigators at the Stanford Heart Disease Prevention Program[40] have compiled a list of six behavioral changes recommended for improved cardiovascular health:

1. Cessation of cigarette smoking
2. Restriction of caloric intake to reach or maintain optimal weight
3. Adjustment of eating habits to reduce intake of saturated fats, cholesterol, simple carbohydrates and salt to reduce serum cholesterol, hypertension, and hyperlipidemia
4. Compliance with drug regimens to control hypertension and hyperlipidemia
5. Acquisition of stress management skills needed to avoid a type A, coronary-prone life-style
6. Establishment of regular physical exercise habits to promote cardiovascular fitness and avoid overweight

The health benefits of these recommended behavioral changes are better documented for disease-free populations than for persons with existing cardiovascular disease. Most research identifying behavioral risk factors or investigating the benefits of such change(s) have in fact been in the area of primary prevention. Investigators have chiefly sought to predict and thereby prevent new disease. Fewer studies have attempted to assess the behavioral risks and benefits of behavioral change among individuals with manifest disease and/or episodes of illness, for example, myocardial infarction. For certain risk factors, including cigarette smoking and the type A behavior pattern, it has been noted that the individual's behavior remains predictive of coronary disease morbidity and mortality even among persons with documented disease.[30,44] In fewer cases, postinfarction changes in behavior have been related to subsequent disease and death. However, two exceptions are noteworthy. Regarding smoking, both Wilhelmsson et al.[60] and Mulcahy et al.[43] studied the secondary prevention value of cessation. The former study found that smokers surviving a first infarction who stopped smoking had only 50% of the rate of recurrence and/or death of those persons who continued to smoke. Similarly, the latter study found that cessation and/or marked reduction in smoking significantly improved the 5-year survival rates of persons experiencing their first infarction. Likewise, a study by Bruce et al.[7] indicates that adherence to a medically supervised exercise program can delay instances of reinfarction among coronary patients.

However, in light of the relative scarcity of findings regarding secondary prevention aspects of behavioral or life-style change among coronary patients, it seems appropriate at this point for health care providers as well as patients to adopt a "Moi Sui" approach to secondary prevention. This approach is outlined in the Canadian government's working document on behavioral risk factors in disease as follows[34]:

> But many of Canada's health problems are sufficiently pressing that action has to be taken on them even if all the scientific evidence is not in. The Chinese have an expression, "Moi Sui" . . . which means "to touch, to feel, to grope around." It reflects a deliberate approach to innovative and creative action even when scientific certainty and predictability are in question.

The emphasis here would be on *taking positive action*, regarding the possible life-saving therapeutic effect(s) of life-style change, rather than focusing entirely on the fact that much more research remains to be done before we can prove the actual benefits of same.

EDUCATIONAL APPROACHES TO RISK REDUCTION

Educational approaches to behavioral risk reduction have prevailed in the health care sector. Such approaches are based on the assumption that the primary determinants of behavior are cognitive and attitudinal and that the *rational* person will give up "bad habits" on being informed about the relative risks involved for coronary disease.

Research has consistently challenged this view of human motivation. Cognitive and attitudinal factors have been shown to play an important, although by no means exclusive, role in motivating and maintaining life-style changes. Literally hundreds of studies[22] have shown that health education, whether through impersonal mass media programming or through interpersonal channels (including physician advice within the context of the doctor-patient relationship) is simply not sufficient by itself to produce desired changes in health behavior. Rather, health education seems to be an essential first step in risk reduction programs, having its greatest impact through enhancing motivation for behavioral change efforts.

Given the critical role of health education in motivating efforts to change behavior, several comments about effective health education for coronary patients seem warranted. As Kasl's[31] "health-belief model" predicts, motivation for behavioral change to prevent disease is a joint function of the perceived threat of (or personal vulnerability to) disease itself and the anticipated "cost and benefits" of the recommended change(s). As such, coronary patients would seem to have a unique susceptibility to educational approaches because of their sense of vulnerability and mortality. This keen sense of perceived threat of disease has, for example, been used to explain the higher quit rates of postinfarction patients, as compared with preinfarction persons, for cigarette smoking.[26] It has also been noted in explaining the finding that wives of coronary patients demonstrate only negligible behavioral change regarding smoking when compared with their recently ill husbands, despite the fact that they were just as well-informed (educated) about the risk of continuing such behavior.[9] In short, the postinfarction patients are usually well aware of the "costs" of failing to become actively involved in risk reduction activities. Health education, on the other hand, could provide for the patient a clear appreciation of the actual "benefits" resulting from such activities. Such educational programs would of necessity need to be *current* regarding research on secondary prevention and *sufficiently broad* to cover all the risk factors: smoking, noncompliance with medication regimen, overweight, excessive caloric and saturated fat intake, and so forth.

BEHAVIORAL APPROACHES TO RISK REDUCTION

Behavioral approaches, as defined in this chapter, refer to *behavior modification* techniques for life-style change that are based on the application of psychological learning theory to altering human behavior. Whereas educational approaches emphasize the cognitive determinants of behavior (habits) and the role of personal choice in behavioral change, behavior modification approaches focus on providing not just the knowledge and motivation for change, but more importantly the skills necessary to achieve such change(s). Behavioral approaches begin by analyzing the behavior in question, for example, smoking, to determine the full range of factors influencing its acquisition and maintenance;

the former is called "response" and the latter "stimuli." Behavioral techniques are aimed at modifying the relationship between stimuli-response factors to make the circumstances less favorable for the development or maintenance of life-threatening habits, while also providing the patient with skills for alternative healthful behaviors, for example, a low-fat diet.

Behavioral approaches use three broad strategies to affect change in life-style: *reinforcement-control, stimulus-control,* and *self-control.* Reinforcement-control involves enhancing motivation to abandon health-threatening behaviors by making the payoffs or consequences for such behaviors less positive for the individual. That is, one might adopt what could be called the "Lysistrata" principle to achieve change(s) in the coronary patient's behavior. The story goes that Lysistrata made the pleasure of her company contingent on (a consequence of) her husband's setting aside the tasks of war. Applied here, the Lysistrata principle suggests using existing social, interpersonal relationships to motivate and reward life-style changes, for example, to make a spouse's approval and affection a consequence of an active physical exercise regimen. Similarly, and in opposite fashion, reinforcement-control can involve punitive or aversive consequences for unwanted, unhealthy behaviors, for example, making the spouse's or friends' social disapproval contingent on smoking.

The second strategy of stimulus-control involves the rearrangement of one's social and physical environment so that one is not led into temptation regarding various bad habits such as overeating. For example, coronary patients who cannot resist attractive, high-calorie foods are instructed not to buy them. If these persons cannot resist buying such foods, they are told to shop for groceries only after a big meal (when food will have less of a natural appeal to them) and/or in stores that do not sell forbidden foods. In such instances, the patient is trained to avoid situations that contain stimuli that traditionally have elicited undesirable behaviors. On the other hand, regarding the problem of hypertension control, such patients may be instructed to develop cues to remind themselves that it is time to take their medication, for example, setting an alarm on their watch or placing the medication to be used at mealtimes on the kitchen table. In short, their task is to engineer an environment that fails to elicit risk behaviors and instead begins to increase the probability of the individual's engaging in antirisk or healthy activities.

The third strategy, often combined with those already discussed, is self-control. This approach primarily involves teaching the individual to be his own behavior modifier as he sees fit, placing most of the responsibility for behavioral change on the patient rather than on other persons, for example, medical and nursing personnel, spouse, and friends. Individuals learn to apply rewards and punishments to themselves as a consequence of certain healthy or unhealthy behaviors in keeping with their understanding of the risks of coronary disease.

They may also learn to develop certain self-cues (which are internal rather than external) that will be instrumental in avoiding unhealthy habits such as noncompliance, such as the thought "It's time to take my medicine."

The rationale behind these various behavioral approaches is summarized elsewhere for the interested reader.[20,40,62] The following description of the various techniques in coronary risk reduction studies perhaps best illustrates their potential use with coronary patients.

Smoking cessation

Broad-spectrum cessation programs. Behavioral research has identified numerous factors, physiological and psychosocial, that contribute to the maintenance of cigarette smoking. These include nicotine dependence, satisfaction from oral, tactile, and respiratory stimulation during the act of smoking, and the role of smoking in the control of stress and anxiety and as an aid to self-expression.[26] Behavioral analyses of the multiple factors, or stimulus conditions, that affect the strength of the smoking habit have pointed out the need for broad-spectrum, multicomponent intervention strategies aimed at a number of factors simultaneously.

Cessation programs based on behavioral analyses of the smoking habit generally involve reducing the probability of smoking by using procedures to make its immediate real or imagined consequences aversive, along with one or more of the following strategies: (1) reinforcing alternatives to smoking behavior (nonsmoking skill training), (2) altering the internal and external stimuli that cue or elicit smoking, and (3) using social influence and support to reinforce smoking behavior change. Weakly effective on their own, these strategies have been found to produce stable outcome in the form of diminished smoking when combined with efforts toward maintaining short-term abstinence.

Aversive procedures. To suppress the smoking response, researchers use punishment (aversive conditioning); in fact, aversive procedures are the mainstay of effective smoking cessation programs. Aversive procedures that use smoke itself as an aversive stimulus are generally more effective than are those that use stimuli unrelated to smoking, for example, electric shock.[3]

The single, most effective smoke aversion technique to date is *rapid smoking,* a procedure in which the person smokes cigarettes only in scheduled laboratory sessions and is instructed to inhale once every 6 seconds for 2 or 3 5-minute trials.[39] Even chronic, heavy smokers find rapid smoking an extremely unpleasant experience, during which they sometimes experience nausea and vomiting. However, even though both short-term and long-term abstinence rates for treatment programs using this procedure have been most impressive,[11] recent research suggests that it may be contraindicated for coronary patients because of potentially hazardous side effects including increased heart rate, blood pressure, and carboxyhemoglobin levels; dizziness; and mild EKG abnormalities.[25,38,42]

On the other hand, research to improve the effectiveness of "safe" smoke aversion alternatives to rapid smoking has provided promising preliminary results. Danaher[10,11] reviews impressive short-term results using a procedure referred to as "regular paced aversive smoking," which involves focusing one's attention on the unpleasant aspects of smoking one's usual cigarettes at normal rates during regularly scheduled laboratory sessions. Kopel[33] reports favorable short-term results with "smoke holding," that is, swishing smoke around in one's mouth without inhaling.

Other smoking suppression alternatives for the coronary patient might involve imagery-based aversive techniques. In one such technique, covert sensitization, smokers imagine (visualize) scenes of extreme nausea and vomiting while smoking and pleasant experiences following termination of such behavior.[8] The effect of techniques that rely on imagery, however, are noticeably less than those that depend on other types of aversive consequences. More research will have to be conducted in this area before such procedures can be reasonably expected to change the overall smoking behavior of coronary patients.

Nonsmoking skill training. The essence of nonsmoking skill training is to equip the ex-smoker with equally satisfying alternatives to the smoking habit. Many programs focus on the role of smoking as a stress management technique and indicate the usefulness of progressive muscle relaxation exercises in this regard.[6] Others focus on substitute oral or manipulative habits that may prove helpful, for example, eating low-calorie foods, chewing on toothpicks or sugarless gum, sucking on hard candies, bending paper clips, or using worry beads.[6,16] Minimal diet counseling may help the neophyte nonsmoker avoid significant weight gain[49] resulting from substitute behaviors. A number of cognitive nonsmoking skills have also been examined including reinforcement of prononsmoking or antismoking thoughts and/or imagining oneself coping without cigarettes in high-anxiety social situations.[6,16]

Environmental or stimulus control. Reducing the frequency and strength of internal and external cues for smoking behavior is the goal of stimulus-control approaches. Common techniques for achieving control over external stimuli that elicit and maintain the smoking of cigarettes seek to narrow the range of situations in which the individual smokes[16] and use a randomly timed signalling device both to cue smoking behavior and to gradually increase the interval between cigarettes. Unfortunately, when stimulus-control techniques are used alone, smokers generally reach a certain minimal level (10 to 14 cigarettes a day) and then gradually return to their pretreatment levels.[3] Using drugs that mimic the effects of nicotine such as lobeline sulfate, small controlled doses of oral nicotine, or minor tranquilizers immediately after cessation to counteract withdrawal effects might be considered under the rubric of stimulus-control aimed at internal control.[3] Though insufficient on their own to produce stable cessation, they may prove of some short-term value as adjuncts to other such strategies.[37]

Social influence and support. Interpersonal factors aiding smoking cessation efforts range from nonspecific effects of a warm, encouraging relationship with the therapist and/or group members[35,39] to the focused use of social reinforcement for behavioral change, as with contingency contracting using friends and family members (the Lysistrata principle).[16,35] Available research indicates that therapist and group support may be more beneficial early, as opposed to later on, in treatment and is best faded out and replaced with self-reinforcement.[3]

The extent of change from broad-spectrum programs. Multicomponent programs have compared favorably with antismoking clinics and other traditional and self-help efforts that typically produce 1-year abstinence rates in the 15% to 21% range.[26] For example, Lando[35] achieved 100% end-of-treatment abstinence and 40% at 6-month follow-up using a broad-spectrum program combining smoke aversion and contingency contracting. Adding booster sessions as well as group contact and social support increased the 6-month abstinence rates to 76%. Studies reviewed by Bernstein and McAlister[3] combined stimulus-control, aversive procedures, and group support to obtain a 1-year abstinence rate of 64% on the average.

Maintenance of behavior change. Maintaining short-term changes in smoking behavior for even 3 months proves difficult to achieve.[27] Maintenance strategies that have looked at long-term effectiveness include therapist follow-up contact,[35] co-participant follow-up using a "buddy system,"[28] and use of prerecorded, encouraging telephone messages.[49] Only therapist contact has proved ineffective, perhaps because it leads clients to attribute their success at cessation to the therapist rather than to themselves. Promising maintenance strategies that have not been systematically studied include ad lib booster sessions,[35] individual counseling to formulate plans to avoid relapse,[37] and cognitive "innoculation" against possible rationalizations for relapse.[11]

Obesity

Most instances of human obesity result from food intake in excess of the demands of energy expenditure required of the individual. Overeating and underexercising are both behaviors that are subject to environmental control. By far the most effective weight control strategies are those based on operant learning theory, for example, those that involve achieving discriminative stimulus-control over eating/exercise behavior and/or involve manipulating reinforcement of these behaviors. As for smoking, multicomponent approaches are most effective.

Self-control and stimulus-control procedures. Self-control and stimulus-control techniques are the mainstay of effective treatment programs for obesity.

Basically, these programs are centered around attempts at teaching individuals to eliminate or suppress both the internal and external stimuli (desire) that trigger eating. Such strategies were first formulated by Ferster et al.[15] and subsequently incorporated by Stuart and Davis[53] in a comprehensive weight reduction program. The intuitive and a priori scientific appeal of these techniques was enhanced by research findings in the late 1960s showing that the eating behavior of obese individuals, more than that of nonobese persons, was highly susceptible to external stimuli such as the proximity, appearance, aroma, visibility, and taste of foods. Common strategies for reducing obesity included:

1. Limiting the number of situations in which eating occurs to lessen situational cues for eating behavior
2. Making unhealthy foods inaccessible, inconspicuous, or difficult to prepare
3. Making small portions of food appear large and eating slowly to heighten satiation
4. Avoiding or weakening internal cues that appear to trigger eating in excess—hunger resulting from food deprivation, boredom, and anxiety

The landmark study using these stimulus-control and self-control techniques in the treatment of obesity was reported by Stuart[52] in 1967; it represented a major breakthrough in this area of intervention. He began with ten overweight women, eight of whom continued until the end of treatment. All the individuals lost more than 20 pounds, and 30% of them lost more than 40 pounds at the end of between 19 and 41 30-minute sessions over a 1-year period. These rates compared favorably with baseline rates established for medical and self-help treatment strategies that cited 20-pound losses for 25% to 28% of subjects and 40-pound losses for only 5% to 8% of obese individuals.[26,55] These rates were also impressive because this type of treatment resulted in a much smaller dropout rate than in nonbehavioral approaches to weight reduction.

The early promise of these techniques to produce consistent short-term losses has not faltered. Weight losses of at least 1 pound per week have resulted from virtually all multicomponent individual or group treatment packages that include them as essential ingredients.[5,29] Most such programs offer the obese patient 8 to 12 weekly sessions followed by booster (follow-up) sessions extending from 6 to 12 months after onset of treatment.

Adjunctive techniques. Rarely are stimulus-control and self-control techniques used alone. In fact, according to a recent review by Stunkard and Mahoney,[54] the most reliably effective treatments are those that combine stimulus-control and self-control techniques with one or more of the following:

1. Self-monitoring or weight-related eating and exercise behaviors and realistic goal-setting
2. Nutritional counseling emphasizing a long-term nutritional exchange strategy, as opposed to short-term restrictive dieting

3. Exercise counseling emphasizing maximally convenient increases in energy output
4. Increasing self-reinforcement for altered eating and exercise behaviors
5. Training those in one's immediate social environment to cue and reinforce behavior change
6. Training in effective alternatives, such as relaxation training, to eating, where it is viewed as a means of controlling stress

Techniques that do not appear to hold much success for effective reduction of weight in obese persons include aversive methods such as covert sensitization (imagining aversive consequences to overeating) and contingency contracting that emphasizes externally mediated, often nonsocial, rewards for short-term changes in weight.[48]

Maintaining short-term losses. Three recent reviews of studies with long-term follow-up data show substantial, although variable, maintenance of short-term weight losses.[5,29,54] It is likely, as with the nonbehavioral approaches, that the end of treatment represents for many patients the end of strong external cues and reinforcers for behavior change. Thus the development of innovative strategies to enhance and prolong treatment impact discussed above is needed if the "fruits of such labor" are to be truly realized.

The coronary-prone (type A) behavior pattern

The behavior of type A individuals (see Chapter 1) is characterized by a hard-driving, competitive pursuit of self-selected goals, chronic impatience, hounding sense of time urgency, excessive job involvement, overengagement in efforts to master (control) environmental challenges, and inability to relax without experiencing guilt and anxiety. The type A individual seems more of a "human doing" than a "human being." Also characteristic of the type A individual is a rigid adherence to the coronary-prone behavior pattern even in the face of expressed desires to change it resulting from primary or secondary concerns about coronary illness.

Analysis of the reinforcers for type A behavior(s) helps explain its rigidity and resistance to change and serves to guide behavior modifiers in their efforts to alter this pathogenic life-style. Two factors have thus far been emphasized:[57] (1) type A behavior is reinforced in a wide variety of settings because it produces outcomes valued by society, for example, money, power, status, and (2) stress plays a key role in maintaining the type A pattern. Regarding the former, social- and self-reinforcement for "nose-to-the-grindstone" behavior are all too common. Regarding the latter, Suinn[57] has outlined a "vicious circle of stress" underlying type A behavior, whereupon individuals respond to the stresses of everyday life with their most familiar coping/mastery behaviors, for example, overscheduling appointments, setting self-imposed deadlines, and exhibiting single-minded pursuit of the tasks at hand. Such behaviors are highly rewarded because they "get the job done" and because they, at least temporarily, alleviate feelings of tension. In the long run, however, these exact same behaviors are stress-producing, leading to the vicious cycle just mentioned. Most behavioral change efforts in this area have been focused on equipping the type A person with alternative, effective stress management techniques.

Stress management training. Suinn and Bloom[58] and Roskies et al.[47] have reported successful attempts to alter type A behavior in middle-aged, male volunteers who are free from symptoms of coronary disease. Their treatment programs consisted primarily of training persons in methods of deep muscle relaxation, teaching them breathing exercises that elicit relaxation, and helping them develop alternative coping strategies for handling everyday stress (which is first visualized and then put into practice). Treatment usually lasts for only 6 to 14 sessions. In both studies, stress management training produced significant improvement in certain type A characteristics, for example, the hard-driving factor, and also in several stress-related psychological traits such as self-reported anxiety and life dissatisfaction. This was true either when type A persons receiving treatment were compared with control persons who did not receive treatment or when their posttreatment levels were compared with pretreatment, baseline measures. In addition, Roskies et al.[47] observed significant changes (decreases) in systolic blood pressure and serum cholesterol levels resulting from this type of therapy, which were apparently unrelated to changes in diet, smoking, or exercise habits. Finally, it was noted that brief group psychotherapy was just as effective in producing healthful changes in type A persons, suggesting that behavioral therapy might not be the only treatment strategy available.[47]

Suinn[56,57] has successfully applied similar stress or anxiety management training to postinfarction outpatients undergoing cardiac rehabilitation as one part of a multicomponent stress management program. A number of other stress management techniques were included: guidance in choosing direct (yoga, meditation, massage) and indirect (music, movies, sports) adjuncts to muscle relaxation, sensitization in bodily cues of stress/tension, identifying various external events that trigger anxiety (traffic jams, interruptions by others, tardiness) and reducing their frequency of occurrence, identifying and learning to control self-generated cues for anxiety (worries about competition and deadlines), and so forth. He reports modest success in altering (by means of self-reports) type A behavior in these patients and also of reducing somewhat their cholesterol and triglyceride levels.

Other methods of stress management for type A persons that use biofeedback and meditation have been suggested by McAlister et al.[40]

Operant approaches to modifying type A behavior. Operant conditioning approaches to type A behavior, also pioneered by Suinn,[56] involve shaping and reinforcing equally productive, though less stress-provoking, behavior in the coronary-prone individual. Examples include using supervisors to set one's priorities, rather than overextending one's commitments, working on demanding tasks only during the most productive times of the day, preventing unnecessary interruptions, removing from view reminders of unfinished work unrelated to the task at hand, cutting down one's daily schedule of activities, screening telephone calls, avoiding meetings with persons who waste time, increasing leisure time activities, and penalizing oneself for impatience.[18,56,57] These life-style "re-engineering" techniques are needed adjuncts to stress management training, which by itself may not be sufficient in the long run unless one learns to change those aspects of the environment that precipitate stress and the resulting type A coping style. Others such as spouses, friends, and employers, will also have to become involved in change efforts if the type A person is to successfully alter these unhealthy habits.

Compliance with prescribed dietary and medical regimens

Even those coronary patients who are highly motivated to follow through with prescribed dietary and medication regimens and who are convinced of their beneficial health consequences experience difficulties achieving desired compliance levels. Ackerman,[1] for example, found that compliance with a low-cholesterol diet among coronary patients dropped from 72% immediately after diet counseling to only 56% 1 year later and, further, that patients' intention and motivation to comply were unrelated to actual compliance. Recent estimates place the national rate of noncompliance with antihypertensive drug regimens at 50%.[26] Noncompliance is not unique to coronary patients, but is widespread and considered by some to be the most important issue facing modern medicine.[20]

In cases in which the patient has adequate knowledge of the prescribed regimen(s) and their benefits, the primary determinants of whether or not compliance occurs are situational. They are related chiefly to the characteristics of the regimen, especially the complexity of the change(s) required in one's daily routine and the strength and consistency of cues (reminders) and reinforcers for complying. Behavioral analysis assumes that compliance is primarily a function of the internal (physical and cognitive cues) and external (environmental) events that precede and immediately follow such behavior.[20,62] In many therapeutic regimens, symptoms (stomach upset) are the natural cues for compliance (take an antacid tablet, avoid spicy foods), and symptom relief (relief from pain and discomfort) is a reinforcer for compliant behavior. In those preventive regimens in which noncompliance is a major problem, for example, hypertension, it is clear that the behaviors required of the patient are indeed quite complex and very often the natural cues and rewards for compliance are absent; that is, there may be no symptoms or symptom relief associated with taking one's medication or staying on a therapeutic diet. Behavioral treatment approaches to problems of compliance attempt to simplify the regimens in question and also to build in substitute cues and reinforcers.

Compliance with dietary regimen. Three dietary changes are typically recommended for coronary patients, as well as for those individuals at risk for coronary disease, that lead to decreases in serum cholesterol and triglyceride levels: (1) limiting overall fat intake to 30% of the total calories and raising the ratio of polyunsaturated/saturated fats; (2) reducing cholesterol intake about 50% to 300 to 350 mg daily, and (3) limiting the intake of sugar so that the ratio of complex carbohydrates to sugar is approximately 3:1.[40,41,50,59] A fourth change, the restriction of daily salt consumption to no more than 3 gm, is often advised for the control of hypertension.

Some of the dietary regimens prescribed to achieve these changes, such as the Stanford Food Plan[41] or the "Help Your Heart Eating Plan,"[21] aim both at lowering blood cholesterol/triglyceride levels and also limiting caloric intake to achieve weight loss. These plans basically involve substituting poultry and fish for beef and fat-marbled meats, limiting egg consumption, substituting polyunsaturated for saturated fats, choosing only low-fat dairy products, and so forth. They also usually require (teach patients) new ways of preparing foods such as broiling versus frying.

Diet counseling is part of most successful programs[41,50] and typically includes modeling of new shopping habits, cooking and dining-out behaviors, and teaching patients about low-cost, available, and enjoyable substitutes for "forbidden" foods, for example, substituting margarine for butter. Behavioral strategies used in conjunction with counseling include cutting down on the "costs" of compliance behavior by simplifying regimens through a step-by-step process and/or reducing economic costs,[41] programming social reinforcement and self-rewards for compliance when dietary changes produce no immediate, natural symptom improvement,[40,41,50] self-monitoring and feedback based on an analysis of diet records or laboratory test results,[40,41,50] and arranging for stimulus-control by using some of the same methods applied to dietary change for weight loss (see section on Obesity). Combined tactics have proved effective in modifying food intake and cholesterol levels.[40,51] Maintaining such changes requires the continuation of effective stimulus-control and reinforcement-control efforts.

Compliance with prescribed drug regimens. Compliance with medication regimens among coronary patients is especially important regarding control of high blood pressure as well as in certain cases requiring control of serum cholesterol levels. Noncompliance is equally problematic for prevention programs aimed at hypertensive and hypercholesteremic conditions because of the punishing, aversive side effects that are not often offset by the rewards of symptom relief.[40] The latter, as noted earlier, is often nonexistent or is long-term and abstract, that is, medication will prevent the onset of further illness and mean better health.

Stimulus-control and reinforcement-control techniques, as well as efforts at simplifying the regimen in question, are effective with drug-taking behavior in the same way they are with diet-adhering behavior. Zifferblatt[62] provides ample guidelines for stimulus-control, suggesting that the best reminders or cues for medication are those that are *salient* (conspicuous and important to the patient), *compatible* with the patient's daily routine, *explicit* or clearly related only to taking drugs, and well-timed so that the *latency* between the cue and taking the drug is short. Examples of good cues include placing prescribed drugs on the dining room table if they are to be taken with meals and using timed, signalling devices or compliance packs and pill calendars that have proved effective in ensuring better compliance. Regimen simplification generally consists of gradually approaching the final, desired dose conditions in a step-by-step fashion.[12,61]

Providing clear social and material reinforcement for compliance has also proved helpful for patients. Wingerson[61] used contingency contracting whereby the patients received cash rewards for compliance. The drug contract also required that the physician prescribe the smallest dose possible, that the physician discuss problems over the phone with the patients, and that long waiting lines for regular check-ups were to be avoided. Paraprofessional health providers have also proved effective in increasing compliance behavior. Haynes et al.[23] found that self-monitoring of blood pressure combined with self-charting of pill-taking behavior and blood pressure along with reinforcement for compliance by a paraprofessional on a schedule every 2 weeks led to a 21.3% increase in compliance and a 30% improvement in blood pressure control after only 6 months. Pharmacists have successfully been involved in similar programs.[61] Ultimately, family and self-reinforcement, however, needs to replace the influence of such external agents if compliance is to be maintained in the absence of prolonged health care contact.

Adherence to physical exercise regimen

Most research evaluating behavioral approaches to promoting adherence to physical exercise regimens has thus far focused on preventive programs geared toward increasing regular or leisure time activity among precoronary volunteers.[13,24,40] There has been less effort to design and evaluate systematic behavioral approaches for promoting such behavior among patients who have suffered myocardial infarctions and other forms of coronary disease. Such programs usually involve two or three weekly group sessions, 45 to 60 minutes in duration, that consist of a walk-jog, calisthenics, and team sport (volleyball, badminton) sequence. Not only are exercise programs tailored to individual medical needs, but all patients begin at low levels of exercise with continual evaluation of physical status determining the rate of progression through the increasingly intensive program.[7,17]

Documented benefits from such programs for coronary patients include improved hemodynamic and functional changes, increased exercise capacity, delay of reinfarction, and improvement in related risk factors such as blood pressure, weight, and cholesterol levels.[7,17,19] Generalizing from findings of precoronary volunteers, one can also expect psychological benefits such as an improved work performance, a greater ability to cope with daily stress, a more positive self-image, and more positive feelings about one's health status.[24] Both the physical and psychological benefits, however, are proportional to the degree of adherence.

Reinforcing adherence. Nonadherence rates for prescribed and supervised exercise programs are notoriously high, with 60% dropout rates not uncommon.[7] Promoting adherence is largely a matter of boosting positive incentives for participation. Data from precoronary volunteers suggest that the most rewarding features of exercise programs involve the social and recreational aspects more than the health and physical fitness benefits.[24] Although the latter may in fact play a more important role in the survival and good health of the individual, it is the camaraderie and variety of activities that most appeals to the patient and keeps him involved in the program. Heinzelman and Bagley[24] also found the adherence behavior of married men to exercise programs to be directly related to their wives' attitude about the program. Poorer adherence occurred when wives were negative, neutral, or indifferent about their husbands' compliance with the exercise regimen. Reinforcement of compliant behavior by significant others would thus be expected to greatly enhance prolonged participation in such programs. In addition, Epstein et al.[13] have stressed the importance of material incentives such as instituting tangible rewards for attendance and degree of involvement. Finally, simply reshaping one's daily routine to include more physical activity such as substituting stairs for escalators or elevators can be most helpful in maintaining achieved cardiovascular fitness.[53]

Self-monitoring and/or medical monitoring. For postinfarction patients, self-monitoring through daily records of symptoms and performance together with frequent medical monitoring[7] would not only provide opportunities for self-reinforcement and social reinforcement (from the medical and nursing personnel) but would also provide needed assurance for common fears about the physical consequences of overexertion such as reinfarction and death. Such fears must always be assessed and dealt with fully by professional care-givers, lest they serve to inhibit adherence to exercise regimens. Medical supervision thus may both provide safeguards for the patients' health and serve as an additional (external) source of motivation and reinforcement.

Research examining systematic efforts to improve adherence in cardiac rehabilitation exercise programs is greatly needed. Increasing exercise demands have proved difficult even with highly motivated, well individuals for whom possible or feared aversive consequences are minimal, not to mention those ill and recuperating individuals for whom such activities have the greatest potential benefit.

MULTIPLE RISK FACTOR REDUCTION

Several treatment programs whose goal it is to reduce cardiovascular risk in coronary patients have sought to achieve multiple life-style changes simultaneously in such individuals. These programs have achieved considerable success in this regard, and their success has suggested that persons who are active in one particular aspect of rehabilitation will also be equally motivated toward changing other risk behaviors in an all-out effort to ensure relative health and survival. Meyer and Henderson[41] and Farquahr et al.[14] of the Stanford Heart Disease Prevention Program have developed, implemented, and evaluated a 10 to 12 week intensive group treatment program for healthy middle-aged men identified as at-risk for coronary disease. Health education along with behavioral treatment techniques are applied to achieve desired changes in the person's diet, smoking habits, serum lipids, weight, blood pressure, and exercise habits—all at the same time. In one instance,[14] treatment efforts were delivered on a community-wide basis by way of an 18-month mass media campaign. Here, as with spouse involvement on the individual patient level, community programming involved the use of group social support as a key element in influencing behavioral change.

Meyer and Henderson[41] found that counseling plus behavioral skills training led to significant and immediate improvements in diet, weight, cholesterol and triglyceride levels, and smoking (except for cigarettes). These improvements were maintained over a 3-month period of follow-up. Only the level of physical exercise was refractory to change. Comparisons of this multiple risk factor approach with one-time physician consultation and also with extended individual counseling indicated that the combined counseling-behavioral approach was definitely superior. Farquahr et al.[14] found that community health education plus intensive face-to-face counseling/behavioral skills training produced marked improvements in smoking rates, dietary intake of cholesterol and saturated fats, plasma lipids, and systolic blood pressure when compared with mass media programming or no treatment. Changes noted in the first year of this program not only persisted through the second follow-up year, they also continued to increase in the desired direction. Other programs designed along similar lines are currently being evaluated for their effect on individuals who have not as yet shown evidence of coronary disease.[32]

Group treatment for the coronary patient and his spouse has also received less attention than one would wish to see. One exception is the report by Rahe et al.[46] in which coronary patients were given 18 hours of group psychotherapy, combined with individualized diet counseling, development of appropriate exercise habits, and advice about smoking cessation. Special attention was given to the so-called "psychological risk factors," including overwork, job dissatisfaction, marital problems, and feelings of time urgency (see Type A behavior pattern). Long-term follow-up of this therapy program indicates that coronary patients receiving treatment, as compared with those not receiving such treatment, had much lower reinfarction rates.[45] Rates of rehospitalization for coronary or bypass surgery and coronary mortality figures were also more positive for the treatment group, although none of these differences reached statistical significance.

SUMMARY

Behavioral approaches aimed at reducing coronary risk factors such as cigarette smoking, obesity, type A behavior pattern, lack of physical exercise, and noncompliance with medication intake (for example, for hypertension control) have to date achieved much success. However, the bulk of the research documenting behavioral change in these areas has been reported for precoronary individuals rather than postcoronary persons (for example, those suffering a myocardial infarction). The latter group of patients should certainly be motivated for change in view of the consequences of not altering their unhealthy habits—death, recurrence of coronary disease, impaired daily function. It is important that patients learn to reward themselves for behavioral change (for example, in their diet or exercise habits) and also to incorporate the reinforcement of significant others in their immediate environment for successful efforts in this regard. Long-term maintenance of behavioral change and life-style modification requires that the individual not solely depend on external factors for motivation. The most effective behavioral programs are those that combine behavioral skills training with health education (for example, mass media), counseling, and psychotherapy to address psychological issues that may interfere with behavioral change in various areas. Multiple risk factor reduction programs are considered promising because individuals who are willing to alter one aspect of their life-style are also generally willing to alter other behaviors that place them at risk for further illness.

REFERENCES

1. Ackerman, A. M.: Factors influencing patient compliance in patients with ischemic heart disease. In Abbott, E. C., et al., editors: A workshop/symposium on compliance, Hamilton, Ontario, Canada, 1977, McMaster University Medical Center.
2. American Heart Association: Report of the Intersociety Commission for Heart Disease Resources, Circulation **42:**A55, 1970.
3. Berstein, D. A., and McAlister, A.: The modification of smoking behavior: progress and problems, Addict. Behav. **1:**89, 1976.
4. Blackburn, H.: Progress in epidemiology and preventing coronary heart disease. In Yu, P., and Goodwin, J., editors: Progress in cardiology, Philadelphia, 1974, Lea & Febriger.
5. Brightwell, D. R., and Sloan, C. L.: Long-term results of behavior therapy for obesity, Behav. Ther. **8:**898, 1977.
6. Brockway, B. S., et al.: Nonaversive procedures and their effects on cigarette smoking, Addict. Behav. **2:**121, 1977.
7. Bruce, E. H., et al.: Comparison of active participants and dropouts in CAPRI cardiopulmonary rehabilitation programs, Am. J. Cardiol. **37:**53, 1976.

8. Conway, J. B.: Behavioral self-control through aversive conditioning and self-management, J. Consult. Clin. Psychol. **45:**348, 1977.
9. Croog, S. H., and Richards, N. P.: Health beliefs and smoking patterns in heart patients and their wives: a longitudinal study, Am. J. Public Health **67:**921, 1977.
10. Danaher, B. G.: Behavioral approaches to smoking cessation. Paper presented at the Annual Meeting of the American Psychological Association, San Francisco, 1977.
11. Danaher, B. G.: Research on rapid smoking: interim summary and recommendations, Addict. Behav. **2:**151, 1977.
12. Dunbar, J., Marshall, G., and Howell, M.: Improving compliance behavioral strategies. In Abbott, E. C., et al., editors: A workshop/symposium on compliance, Hamilton, Ontario, Canada, 1977, McMaster University Medical Center.
13. Epstein, L. H., Thompson, J. K., and Griffin, W.: Compliance and fitness in two aerobics exercise programs. Cited in Epstein, L. H., and Cincirpini, P. M.: Behavior medicine III: health care delivery, Assoc. Advance. Behav. Ther. Newsletter **4:**7, 1977.
14. Farquhar, J. W., et al.: Community education for cardiovascular health, Lancet **1:**1192, 1977.
15. Ferster, C. B., Nurnberger, J. J., and Levitt, E. B.: The control of eating, J. Math. **1:**87, 1962.
16. Flaxman, J.: Quitting smoking now or later: gradual, abrupt, immediate and delayed quitting, Behav. Ther. **9:**260, 1978.
17. Fletcher, G. F., and Cantwell, J. D.: Outpatient gym exercise program for patients with recent myocardial infarction, Arch. Intern. Med. **134:**63, 1974.
18. Friedman, M., and Rosenman, R. H.: Type A behavior and your heart, Greenwich, Conn., 1974, Fawcett Publishing Co.
19. Froelicher, V. F., and Oberman, A.: Analysis of epidemiological studies of physical inactivity as risk factor for coronary artery disease, Prog. Cardiovasc. Dis. **15:**41, 1972.
20. Gentry, W. D.: Noncompliance to medical regimen. In Williams, R. B., and Gentry, W. D., editors: Behavioral approaches to medical treatment, Cambridge, Mass., 1977, Ballinger Publishing Co.
21. Gotto, A. M., et al.: HELP your heart eating plan, Houston, 1975, Baylor College of Medicine.
22. Green, L. W.: Diffusion and adoption of innovations related to cardiovascular risk behavior in the public. In Enelow, A. J., and Henderson, J. B., editors: Applying behavioral science to cardiovascular risk, Dallas, 1975, American Heart Association.
23. Haynes, R. B., et al.: Improvement of medication compliance in uncontrolled hypertension, Lancet **1:**1265, 1976.
24. Heinzelman, R., and Bagley, R. W.: Response to physical activity programs and their effects on health behavior, Public Health Rep. **85:**905, 1970.
25. Horan, J. J., et al.: Rapid smoking: a cautionary note, J. Consult. Clin. Psychol. **45:** 341, 1977.
26. Houpt, J., et al.: Relationship of health to general health care, Washington, D.C., 1977, Institute of Medicine, National Academy of Sciences.
27. Hunt, W. A., and Bespalec, D. A.: An evaluation of current methods of modifying smoking behavior, J. Clin. Psychol. **30:**431, 1974.
28. Janis, I. L., and Hoffman, D.: Facilitating effects of daily contact between partners who make decision to stop smoking, J. Pers. Soc. Psychol. **17:**25, 1970.
29. Jeffrey, R. W., Wing, R. R., and Stunkard, A. J.: Behavioral treatment of obesity: the state of the art 1976, Behav. Ther. **9:**189, 1978.
30. Jenkins, C. D.: The coronary-prone personality. In Gentry, W. D., and Williams, R. B., editors: Psychological aspects of myocardial infarction and coronary care, ed. 2, St. Louis, 1979, The C. V. Mosby Co.
31. Kasl, S. V.: Social psychological characteristics associated with behaviors which reduce cardiovascular risk. In Enelow, A. J., and Henderson, J. B., editors: Applying behavioral science to cardiovascular risk, Dallas, 1975, American Heart Association.
32. Kolata, G. B.: Prevention of heart disease: clinical trials at what cost? Science **190:**764, 1975.
33. Kopel, S.: Paper presented at the Annual Meeting of the Association for Advancement of Behavior Therapy, Atlanta, 1977.
34. Lalonde, M.: A new perspective on the health of Canadians, Ottawa, 1974, Ministry of National Health and Welfare.

35. Lando, H.: Successful treatment of smokers with a broad-spectrum behavioral approach, J. Consult. Clin. Psychol. **45:**361, 1977.
36. Levitz, L. S., and Stunkard, A. J.: A therapeutic coalition for obesity: behavior modification and patient self-help, Am. J. Psychiatry **131:**423, 1974.
37. Lichtenstein, E., and Danaher, B. G.: Role of the physician in smoking cessation. In Brashear, R. E., and Rhodes, M. L., editors: Chronic obstructive lung disease: clinical treatment and management, St. Louis, 1978, The C. V. Mosby Co.
38. Lichtenstein, E., and Glascow, R. E.: Rapid smoking: side effects and safeguards, J. Consult. Clin. Psychol. **45:**815, 1977.
39. Lichtenstein, E., et al.: Comparison of rapid smoking, warm smoky air and attention placebo in the modification of smoking behavior, J. Consult. Clin. Psychol. **40:**92, 1973.
40. McAlister, A. L., et al.: Behavioral science applied to cardiovascular health: progress and research needs in the modification of risk-taking habits in adult population, Health Educ. Monogr. **4:**45, 1976.
41. Meyer, A. J., and Henderson, J. B.: Multiple risk factor reduction in the prevention of cardiovascular disease, Prev. Med. **3:**225, 1974.
42. Miller, L. C., et al.: Potential hazards of rapid smoking as a technic for the modification of smoking behavior, N. Engl. J. Med. **297:**590, 1977.
43. Mulcahy, R., et al.: Factors affecting the 5 year survival rate of men following acute coronary heart disease, Am. Heart J. **93:**556, 1977.
44. NCSH (National Clearinghouse for Smoking and Health): The Health Consequences of Smoking—1975, Atlanta, 1975, U.S. Department of Health, Education, and Welfare.
45. Rahe, R. H.: Brief group therapy for post-myocardial infarction patients: a 3 to 4 year follow-up of a controlled trial. Paper presented at the 35th Annual Meeting of the American Psychosomatic Society, Washington, D.C., 1978.
46. Rahe, R. H., et al.: Group therapy in the outpatient management of post-myocardial infarction patients, Psychiatr. Med. **4:**77, 1973.
47. Roskies, E., et al.: Changing the coronary prone (type A) behavior pattern in a non-clinical population, J. Behav. Med. **1:**201, 1978.
48. Saccone, A. J., and Israel, A. C.: Effects of experimenter versus significant other-controlled reinforcement and choice of target behavior on weight loss, Behav. Ther. **9:**271, 1978.
49. Shewchuk, L. A.: Smoking cessation programs of the American Health Foundation, Prev. Med. **5:**454, 1976.
50. Shorey, R. L., et al.: Alterations of serum lipids in a group of free living adult males, Am. J. Clin. Nutr. **27:**268, 1974.
51. Stamler, J.: Epidemiology of coronary heart disease, Med. Clin. North Am. **57:**5, 1973.
52. Stuart, R. B.: Behavioral control of overeating, Behav. Res. Ther. **5:**357, 1967.
53. Stuart, R. B., and Davis, B.: Slim chance in a fat world: behavioral control of obesity, Champaign, Ill., 1972, Research Press.
54. Stunkard, A. J., and Mahoney, M. J.: Behavioral treatment of eating disorders. In Leitenberg, H., editor: Handbook of behavior modification and behavior therapy, Englewood Cliffs, N.J., 1976, Prentice-Hall, Inc.
55. Stunkard, A. J., and McLaren-Hume, M.: The results of treatment for obesity: a review of the literature and report of a series, Arch. Intern. Med. **125:**1067, 1970.
56. Suinn, R. M.: Behavior therapy for cardiac patients, Behav. Ther. **5:**569, 1974.
57. Suinn, R. M.: Type A behavior pattern. In Williams, R. B., and Gentry, W. D., editors: Behavioral approaches to medical treatment, Cambridge, Mass., 1977, Ballinger Publishing Co.
58. Suinn, R. M., and Bloom, L. J.: Anxiety management training for type A persons, J. Behav. Med. **1:**25, 1978.
59. U.S. Senate Select Committee on Nutrition and Human Needs: Dietary goals for the United States, Washington, D.C., 1977, U.S. Government Printing Office.
60. Wilhelmsson, C., et al.: Smoking and myocardial infarction, Lancet **1:**415, 1975.
61. Wingerson, L.: Hypertension compliance, Med. World News **18:**20, 1977.
62. Zifferblatt, S. M.: Increasing patient compliance through the applied analysis of behavior, Prev. Med. **4:**173, 1975.

Index

A

Achievement, striving for, 13
Activity; *see* Physical activity and rehabilitation
Acute care, 65-110; *see also* Coronary care unit
Alienation and coronary care unit staff, 102; *see also* Stress, coronary care unit nurses and
American Heart Association pamphlets for patient teaching, 161
A.N.A. Standards of Cardiovascular Nursing Practice, 94-96
Angina pectoris, 5
  history of, and delay in seeking medical help, 69-70
  risk factors for, 6
  sexual activity and, 119
  type A behavior and, 25
Anticipation, 161
  art of, instruction in, 158
  preadmission behavior and, 152
Antidepressants, tricyclic, 156, 160
Anxiety, 150; *see also* Coping; Stress
  angina pectoris and, 6-7, 25
  coronary care unit experience and, 152
    psychological intervention and, 152-153
  coronary care unit nurses and, 109
  fight-or-flight activity in response to, 34
  hypnosis as intervention and, 155
  impaired libido and, 120
  medications and, 92-93
  after myocardial infarction, 113
  rehabilitation and, 113; *see also* Rehabilitation
  sexual activity and, 118-120
  spouses of coronary patients and, 98; *see also* Family(ies) of coronary patients; Spouse(s) of coronary patients
Arrest, cardiac; *see* Cardiac arrest
Atheromatous plaque; *see* Atherosclerosis
Atherosclerosis
  hypothalamic stimulation and progression of, 56
  psychosocial factors and, 50-64
  psychosocial stress, experimental, and, 57
  type A behavior and, 8, 50
Augmenting and reducing phenomenon, 58-59
Autohypnosis, 155

B

Balloon pump, intra-aortic, 97-98
B.A.S.I.C. I.D., 138-139
Behavior(s); *see also* Conflict(s); Coping; Stress; specific behaviors and feeling states
  after acute myocardial infarction, 67-77
  avoidance, and cardiovascular responses, 52
  cardiovascular responses and, 53-56
  changes in, 172-173
  coping; *see* Coping
  coronary disease and, summary of possible mediating factors, 60
  of coronary patient; *see* Coronary patient; specific behaviors
  coronary prone, patterns of; *see* Coronary-prone behavior pattern
  denial, 70-71, 84-85
    counterphobic, 115
      drug misuse and, 122
    definition of, 70-71
    delay in seeking medical help and, 70-71
  fight-or-flight activities and, 33-34
    as excitatory response, 34
    hemodynamic responses and, 33
  maladaptive
    counterphobic denial and, 115
    drug misuse and, 122
    invalidism, cardiac, as, 115
    psychological interventions and, 150

Behavior(s)—cont'd
overt, and assessment of coronary-prone behavior pattern, 14
perceptual style and, 58
physiological correlates of, 52-56
preadmission; *see* Preadmission behavior(s)
rehabilitation and, 114-116
as risk factor for coronary disease, 7-14
scapegoating, in coronary care unit, 98, 102, 103-104
sensory intake, 53
changes in forearm vascular resistance during, 53-54
sensory rejection, 53-54
hemodynamic responses and, 55
stereotyping, and coronary care unit nurses, 101-102
type A; *see* Type A behavior(s); Type A individual(s)
type B; *see* Type B behavior(s); Type B individual(s)
Behavior modification techniques, 174
Benzodiazepines, 156, 160
Biofeedback, 61
Blood flow to skeletal muscle, and stress, 52, 53
Blood pressure; *see also* Hypertension
elevated, in response to stress, 52
experimental, hypothalamic stimulation and, 56
lability of, and coronary disease, 55
Breathing and type A and type B behaviors, 20-22

C

Cardiac arrest
denial and, 151-152
emotional effect of, on coronary care unit nurses, 98-99
mechanisms of, 33-35
Cardiac function, 78-89
catecholamines and, 45-46
life events and, 45-46
Cardiac invalidism; *see* Invalidism, cardiac
Cardiac output
fight-or-flight activity and, 56
increased, and avoidance behavior, 52
stress and, 55
Cardiac rehabilitation occupational stress inventory, 143-144
Cardiovascular function; *see also* Cardiovascular system
behavior and, 52-56
central nervous system mechanisms and, 56
Cardiovascular function—cont'd
perceptual style and, 57-59
processing of sensory information and, 58
stress and, experimental findings, 56
sympathetic nervous system and, 57
Cardiovascular system
avoidance behavior and, 52
changes in, and behavioral manipulation, 52-56
sensory intake behavior and, 54
sexual activity and, 119
Catecholamines, 45-46
sensory intake behavior and, 58
stress and, 56
Central nervous system and cardiovascular function, 56; *see also* Sympathetic nervous system
Chest pain, 77, 151
Chlordiazepoxide, 156, 160
Clinical recognition of coronary-prone personality, 14-22
Communication
conflict between coronary care unit staff and other hospital personnel and, 101
nurse-physician, and care of terminal patient, 106-107
patient-physician, 123-124, 125
Community agencies in cardiac rehabilitation, 122-123
Competition as source of stress in coronary care unit, 101, 102
Competitiveness as risk factor for coronary disease, 13
Conflict(s); *see also* Stress
care of terminal patients and, 105-108
in coronary care unit, 106-107
general areas of, 99
group meetings to deal with, 99-101
masking of, 103-105
nurses and, 97
patients as source of, 98-99
in families, after myocardial infarction, 113; *see also* Family(ies) of coronary patients
Confrontation as means of psychological intervention, 152
Contracts, behavior change, 96
Conservation-withdrawal, 34
Convalescence; *see* Rehabilitation
Coping; *see also* Psychological intervention; Stress; specific behaviors and problems
anxiety and; *see* Anxiety
central nervous system and, 56
coronary care unit nurses and, 90-110
group meetings and, 99-101

Coping—cont'd
failure in, 150
fight-or-flight activity, 33-34
maladaptive, 150; *see also* Behavior(s), maladaptive
mechanisms in, 78
perspectives in, 80
psychological, 80
rehabilitation and, 113-130
stress reaction and, 55
Coronary care unit, 81-85
behaviors of type A patients in, 22-24
conflict in, 99; *see also* Stress
general areas of, 99
group meetings and, 99-101
masking of, 103-105
patients as source of, 98-99
role of head nurse in, 104
dying patients as source of stress in, 106-107
equipment in, 91-92, 154-155
hypnosis in, 155
morale of staff in, 109
nursing in, 90-110; *see also* Nurses, coronary care unit
administration, 98, 104-105
bedside learning and, 91
comfort and, 80
competition and, 101
patient perceptions of, 90-91
stress and, 97-98
teaching functions and, 96
orientation of newly admitted patients to, 153-154
patients in; *see* Coronary patients
pecking order in, 102
psychological intervention in, 149-161; *see also* Psychological interventions
staff in, 82-85, 97-108, 155
stereotyping in, 101-102
temporary assignment to, 101-102
terminal patients and, 105-108
treatment compartmentalization in, 83
Coronary disease; *see also* Myocardial infarction
behavior and
mediating factors in, 60
patterns of, as risk factors in, 7-14
blood pressure lability and, 55
clinical subtypes of, and behavior pattern, 25-26
common misconceptions and, 156-157
coronary-prone behavior pattern and; *see* Coronary-prone behavior pattern
etiology of, 3-64; *see also* Risk factors
historical perspectives of, 5-7
Coronary disease—cont'd
etiology of—cont'd
psychological mechanisms and physiological responses and, 50-64
future, and type A behavior, 25
general perspectives of, 1-2
history of, and delay in seeking medical help, 69-70
incidence of, control of risk factors and changes in, 59, 61
individual differences and susceptibility to, 57-59
intervention in, 147-189
Jenkins Activity Survey scores to predict, 10
life events, critical, and, 31-49
cumulative, 39-43
mechanisms linking, 43-44
mortality from, and type A behavior, 13
myths about, 156-157
pathogenesis of, studies in, 6
prevention and treatment of, 59-62
psychosocial factors in, 26
physiological mechanisms and, 50-64
risk factors; *see* Risk factors, for coronary disease
role of individual differences in, 57-59
sex differences in incidence of, 14
type A behavior and; *see* Type A behavior(s); Type A individual(s)
work and; *see* Work
Coronary patient(s), 85-88
actions of, 13
acute care of, 65-110; *see also* Coronary care unit
age of, and delay in seeking medical help, 68, 69
anxiety and; *see* Anxiety
assessment of, and rehabilitation, 124-126
behaviors of, as threat to coronary care unit nurses, 100-101
group meetings to cope with, 99-101
cardiac function in, 78-89
care of, 90-96
characteristics of, 138
community agencies in rehabilitation of, 122-123
confidence of, 154-155
contract with, 96
coping and, 78-89; *see also* Coping
adequacy of, 150
coronary disease history and, 69-70
counterphobic denial by, 115
death of, 103
decision time of, 67-68; *see also* Decision time

Coronary patient(s)—cont'd
deconditioning and, 115, 119-120
denial and; *see* Denial
depression and; *see* Depression
drugs and, common problems with, 120-122; *see also* Medication(s)
emotional reactions of, 114-116
energy expenditure and limitations of, 126
evaluation of, 137
families of; *see* Family(ies) of coronary patients
faulty symptom attribution and, 67, 69
fears of; *see* Fear(s)
functioning of, 137
group therapy and, 61
human contact with, 78-89
illness perception by, 70-71
intervention for, 153-158
invalidism and; *see* Invalidism, cardiac
motivation of, 96
newly admitted, orientation of, 153-154
nontherapeutic activities of, 72-74
nurse teaching and, 96
perceptions of, 90-91
personal needs of, 157
physical activity and, 164-166; *see also* Rehabilitation
physician(s) and
delay in call for, 74-75, 77
relationship of, 123-124
positive reinforcement of, 116
preadmission behaviors of; *see* Preadmission behavior(s)
prolongation of life and, 107
psychological aftermaths of myocardial infarction and, 113-130
psychological characteristics of, 5-6
psychological intervention and, 149-161
preparation for, 149-150
rehabilitation of; *see* Rehabilitation
response of, to coronary care unit nurses, 90-91
self-destructive patterns of, 115
self-esteem of, 158-159
self-treatment by, 72-74
sexual misbehaviors of, 100-101
sexual problems of; *see* Sexual activity; Sexual counseling of coronary patients
social context of symptom onset and response of, 71-72
as source of conflict in coronary care unit, 98-99
speech of, 13
spouses of; *see* Spouse(s) of coronary patients
Coronary patient(s)—cont'd
stages of recovery of, 114-115
symptom interpretation by, 69
terminal care of, 105-108
trust and, 116
type A, and implications for care, 22-24
typical response of, to myocardial infarction, 67-69
as work addicts, 12
work-related conflicts and; *see* Work
Coronary-prone personality, 5-30; *see also* Risk factors; Type A behavior(s); Type A individual(s)
as all-or-none phenomenon, 24
breathing and, 20-22
clinical psychological considerations of, 7
clinical recognition of, 14-22
definition of, 6
effect of, in rehabilitation, 114-116
explanation of, to type A patients, 23
facial expression and, 19-20
gestures and movements and, 19
implications of, for medical care, 22-24
individual differences and, 57-59
at intake, 7-8
intensity of, and proportional risk of coronary disease, 25
origins of concept of, 5-7
personal values associated with, 15-16
as predictor of clinical subtypes of coronary disease, 25
questions about, 24-26
as reflection of socioeconomic status, 24
as risk factor for coronary disease, 24-25
root causes of, 23
as style of behavior, 6
style of thought and, 16
vocational involvement and, 12-13
Western Collaborative Group Study findings and, 7-8
work-related aspects of; *see* Work
Counseling
diet, 183
strategies for, 139-140
Counselor, rehabilitation, 145
Counterphobic denial, 115
CPBP; *see* Coronary-prone behavior pattern
Crisis, normal responses to, 115; *see also* Coping; Stress

D

Dalmane; *see* Flurazepam
Death; *see also* Mortality; Terminal patient(s)
fear of, 91

Death—cont'd
fear of—cont'd
delay in seeking medical help and, 71
impending, nurses' response to, 99
as source of stress to coronary care unit staff, 98-99
sudden, and life events, 41
after traumatic event, 31-33
voodoo, 32
Decision time; *see also* Delay; Preadmission behavior(s)
day of symptom onset and, 73
definition of, 67
demographic factors in, 69
medical, 74-75
perception of illness and, 70-71
of sample group of coronary patients, 68
social context of symptom onset and, 71-72
time of day of symptom onset and, 71-72
Deconditioning
rehabilitation and, 125
sexual activity and, 119-120
Defense mechanisms; *see also* Coping; Denial; Psychological intervention
in coronary care unit, 152-153
forms of, 153
Delay
physician, 74-75, 77
in seeking medical help, 67-77, 151; *see also* Preadmission behavior(s)
demographic characteristics and, 69
perception of illness and, 70-71
psychological intervention, 151-152
social context of symptom onset and, 71-72
socioeconomic variables and, 151
Demographic characteristics
affecting preadmission behaviors, 69
coronary disease and, 24
Denial, 70-71, 84-85; *see also* Coping; Psychological intervention
anxiety and, 152-153
cardiac arrest and, 151-152
conscious, 153
counterphobic, 115
delay in seeking medical help and, 151-152
maximal, 71
minimal, 71
unconscious, 153
Depression, 150, 153, 158
angina pectoris and, 6-7
coronary care unit nurses and, 91, 109
in coronary patients, 93, 113, 152-153
etiology of, 93
nursing intervention and, 93
Depression—cont'd
etiological factors in, 93
homecoming, 159
impaired libido and, 120
medications and, 160
prevention of, 116
psychological intervention, 152
rehabilitation and, 113
type A behavior and susceptibility to, 159
Diazepam, 156, 160
Diet, compliance with, 182-183
Dinnerstein 5 decision, 107
DNR, 106-107
Domestic problems and rehabilitation of coronary patients, 114; *see also* Family(ies) of coronary patients; Spouse(s) of coronary patients
Dopamine-beta-hydroxylase, 57, 58
Doxepin, 160
Drugs; *see* Medication(s)

E

Economic factors in misuse of medications, 121
Education
as means of psychological intervention, 152, 153-154
myocardial infarction symptoms and, 76-77
risk reduction and, 173-174
Ego infarction, 93
healing of, 116
Ejaculation, premature, 162, 163
Electrodyne monitor pacemaker, 154
Emergency room treatment subsequent to myocardial infarction, 152
Emotional response to myocardial infarction, 79-80, 113; *see also* Psychological intervention
Environment, coronary care unit, orientation of patient to, 91-92
Epinephrine and psychological stress, 45
Erection, failure of, 162-163
Etiology of coronary disease, 3-64; *see also* Risk factors
coronary-prone personality and, 5-30
historical perspectives of, 5-7
psychosocial factors, physiological mechanisms and, 50-64
Exercise
physical conditioning and, 159-160
training, 156

F

Facial expression and behavior, 19-20

Family(ies) of coronary patients; *see also* Spouse(s) of coronary patients
anxiety of, staff concern for, 98
conflicts and depression and, 115-116
domestic problems and, 114
emotional conflict in, 113
follow-up telephone calls to, 160
guilt and, 118
involvement in rehabilitation of type A patients, 23-24
patient teaching and, 96
problems with medications and, 121
psychosocial factors and, 125
rehabilitation and, 116-118
role of, in seeking medical help, 71, 76
as source of conflict in coronary care unit, 97
of terminal patient, 99
therapy for, 156-157
FD individuals; *see* Field-dependent individuals
Fear(s)
coronary care unit nurses and, 91
of coronary patients, 91, 152
during recovery, 114-115
medications and, 92-93
spouses of coronary patients and, 116-117
therapeutic rule for treatment of, 92
FI individuals; *see* Field-independent individuals
Field articulation, 58
Field-dependent individuals
cardiovascular responses in, 58
perceptual style of, 58
Field-independent individuals
cardiovascular responses in, 58
perceptual style of, 58
Fight-or-flight activities, 33-34
conservation-withdrawal vs., 34
hemodynamic responses and, 34, 56
as response to anxiety, 34
Float list, 101, 102
Flurazepam, 156
Follow-up telephone calls to patient and family, 160
Fractional anticipatory goal reactions, 16

G

Gestures and type A and type B behavior, 19
Group(s)
meetings of in coronary care unit, 99-101
outpatient, 118
Group therapy, 61, 186-187
Guilt
coronary care unit nurses and, 109
families of coronary patients and, 118

H

Heart clubs, 160
Heart disease; *see* Cardiovascular function; Cardiovascular system; Coronary disease; Risk factors
Historical perspectives on coronary disease, 5-6
Hobbies, resumption of, 133
Hospital arrival time, 67, 68
Hospitalization, 152-158; *see also* Coronary care unit
Hostility, 13-14
coronary care unit nurses and, 109
Hypertension; *see also* Blood pressure
experimentally produced stress and, 56
history of, and delay in seeking medical help, 70
Hypnosis, 155
Hypotension, orthostatic, and deconditioning, 115
Hypothalamus
fight-or-flight activity and, 56
stimulation of ventromedial nucleus of, and atherosclerosis, 56

I

Illness and cumulative life events, 35-39
life events–health change theory of, 35-38
psychosomatic theory of, 35
Infarction, ego, 93
healing of, 116
Inorgasmia, secondary, 163
Instructions for drug use, 121
Intensive care unit; *see* Coronary care unit
Interpersonal relationships, type A and type B behavior and, 16-18
Intervention, 147-189
psychological; *see* Psychological interventions
Invalidism, cardiac, 113-114; *see also* Rehabilitation
onset of, 113
physician and, 115-116
threat of, and depression, 158

J

Jenkins Activity Survey, 7, 8-11
occupational level and high risk scores in, 24
scores of, as predictors of new coronary disease, 10, 21, 25
type A behaviors and coronary disease in, 10
Job analysis, 142

L

Lazarus, B.A.S.I.C. I.D. program of, 138-139
Levarterenol bitartrate, 106-107

Levophed; *see* Levarterenol bitartrate
Libido, impaired, and anxiety and depression, 120
Life Change Units (LCU), 40
  variations in, 44
Life events, critical, 31-49
Lipid metabolism; *see also* Serum cholesterol levels
  hypothalamic stimulation and control of, 56
  individual differences in, related to psychosocial factors, 58-59
  life stresses and, 54
Lobeline sulfate, 177
Locus ceruleus, 56
Loneliness, 86-87

M

Maladaptive behavior(s)
  counterphobic denial and, 115
  drug misuse and, 121
  invalidism, cardiac, as, 115
  psychological interventions in, 150
Medical care
  delay in seeking, 67-77; 151
  of type A patients, 22-24
Medication(s), 92-93, 160
  compliance with, 182-184
  dependence on, 122
  misuse of
    economic factors in, 121
    instructions for use and, 121
    psychosocial factors in, 122
  psychological intervention in rehabilitation and, 155-156
  rehabilitation and, 120-122
  sexual activity and, 120
Men, postcoronary, and sexual dysfunction, 162-163
Methyldopa, 168
Minnesota Multiphasic Personality Inventory, 7
Monitoring equipment, 92
Morale of coronary care unit staff, 109
Mortality and preadmission behavior, 76
Motivation, 173-174
Myocardial infarction; *see also* Coronary disease; Coronary patient(s)
  blood pressure, lowered, and incidence of, 51
  depression subsequent to, 93
  emotional distress and, 113
  emotional reactions to, 79-80
  history of, and delay in seeking medical help, 69-70
  hospital arrival time after, 67
  incidence of sudden death and, 67
Myocardial infarction—cont'd
  medication misuse after, 121
  patient functioning and, 137
  physical activity after, 116
  preadmission behavior(s) and, 67-77
  psychological aftermaths of, 113-130
  psychological intervention and, 149-161
  psychological problems of, phases of, 150
  recovery from, definition of, 127
  recurrent
    perceptual style and risk of, 58
    risk of, and type A behavior, 11, 23
  rehabilitation after; *see* Rehabilitation
  response to symptoms of, 67
    typical, 67-69
  return to work after, 132-133
  risk factors in, 5-7
  sexual problems and, 118-120, 133, 157
  stages of recovery from, 114-115
    life events and, 40
  type A behavior characteristics predictive of, 25
  uncomplicated, 125
  vocational stages and, 140

N

Neuroticism and angina pectoris, 6-7, 25
Neurotransmitters, effect of stress on synthesis of, 57
Nicotine, oral, 177
Nitroglycerin, 165
Norepinephrine
  infusions of, and platelet aggregation, 57
  plasma levels of
    increased, 57
  type A men and, 57
  psychological stress and, 45
Nucleus, ventromedial; *see* Hypothalamus
Nurses, coronary care unit, 90-110; *see also* Coronary care unit, nursing
  ability to listen and, 93
  alienation and, 102
  bedside learning and, 91
  care of, 97-108
  communication among, 101
  competence of, 91
    patient security and, 91
    as source of intrastaff conflict, 101
  competition among, 101, 102
  conflict and, 97
    masking of, 103-105
  desirable characteristics of, 90-91
  divisiveness and, 109
  hazing among, 102-103

Nurses, coronary care unit—cont'd
head, role of in conflict, 104
intervention by, 147-189
lifting by, 97
morale of, 109
needs of, 97-98
newly admitted patients and, 91-92
paranoia and, 104-105
patient care and, 90-96
patient perception of, 90-91
pecking order of, 102
personality patterns of, 84, 109-110
physician communication and, 105
reaction of patients to, 91
reasons for choice of profession and, 109-110
scapegoating and, 98, 102, 103-104
self-esteem of, 101
as source of conflict in coronary care unit, 99
stereotyping behavior of, 101-102
stress and, 101-103
group meeting for, 99-101
staff-created, and, 101-103
successful, characteristics of, 91
teaching functions of, 93-96
terminal patients and
care of, 105-108
treatment plans for, 106

O

Obesity
adjunctive techniques for, 179-180
self-control procedures for, 178-179
short-term losses and, 180
stimulus-control procedures for, 178-179

P

Pain
coronary care nurses and, 97
experience of, 150
Pathogenesis of coronary disease, studies in, 6
Patient, coronary; *see* Coronary patient(s)
Patient teaching
American Heart Association materials for, 161
coronary care unit nurses and, 93-96
goal of, 94
as means of psychological intervention, 153-154
Perception(s)
of illness, 70-71
of symptoms of myocardial infarction, 68-69
Perceptual style, 57-59
augmenting and reducing phenomenon and, 58
Perceptual style—cont'd
cardiovascular responses and, 57-59
differences in, 59
Personality
of coronary care unit nurses, 109-110
coronary-prone; *see* Coronary-prone personality; Type A behavior(s); Type A individual(s)
Phenothiazines, 156, 160
Physical activity and rehabilitation, 159-160
adherence to, 184-186
monitoring of, 185-186
reinforcement of, 185
Physician(s)
adjustment problems in rehabilitation and, 123-124
communication with nurses and, 105
critical qualities in, 123
delay of, and care of coronary patients, 74-75, 77
human traits of, and rehabilitation, 123
patient relationships with, 123-124
role of, in rehabilitation, 123-124
as source of conflict in coronary care unit, 99
Physiological correlates of behavior, 52-56
Physiological mechanisms and psychosocial factors in coronary disease, 50-64
Plaque, atheromatous; *see* Atherosclerosis
Postcoronary patients; *see* Coronary patient(s); Rehabilitation
Preadmission behavior(s), 67-77, 151-152; *see also* Delay
case study of, 151
cognitive functions in decision to seek medical help and, 70
demographic factors and, 69
factors in, 69-72
history of coronary disease and, 69-70
interventions in, 151-152
mortality and, 76
perception of illness and, 70-71
physician delay and, 74-75
psychological interventions and, 151
self-treatment and nontherapeutic activities and, 72-74
social context of symptom onset and, 71-72
Prevention and treatment of coronary disease, 59-62
Propranolol, 61, 165, 168
Psychiatrist and myocardial infarction patients, 149, 152-153
Psychological aftermaths of myocardial infarction, 113-130

Psychological interventions, 61, 149-161; *see also* Coping; Rehabilitation; Stress; specific behaviors and feeling states
  confidence in coronary care unit equipment and staff and, 154-155
  confrontation and, 155
  in coronary care unit, 156-158
  education and explanation and, 153-154
  exercise training and, 156
    physical conditioning and, 159-160
  factors in, 149
  family therapy and, 156-157
  follow-up with patient and family and, 160
  heart clubs and, 160
  hypnosis and, 155
  instruction in art of anticipation and, 158, 161
  medications and, 155-156
  patient preparation for, 149-150
  preadmission behavior and, 151-152
  rehabilitation and, 158-161
  relaxation techniques in, 161
  support and respect for patient's personal needs and, 157-158
Psychosocial factors and coronary disease, 26, 79, 86
  physiological mechanisms and, 50-64
  sexual health and, 164

R

Regression, 150
Rehabilitation, 111-146, 158-161
  assessment of patient and, 124-126
  basis for, 131
  community agencies in, 122-123
  deconditioning and, 115
  definition of, 127
  depression and, 113
    psychological intervention and, 158-161
  domestic problems and, 114; *see also* Family(ies) of coronary patients
  energy expenditures and limitations and, 126
  exercise and, 156
  families, importance in, 116-118
  follow-up telephone calls to patients and families, 160
  general considerations in, 124-126
  group therapy in, 61
  heart clubs and, 160
  individualized physical programs in, 125
  interventions in, 159-161
  invalidism, cardiac, and, 113-114
  maladaptive behaviors and, 115-116
Rehabilitation—cont'd
  medication and, 120-122
    common problems with, 120-122
    sexual activity and, 120
  outcome of, and patient-physician relationship, 123-124
  outpatient groups and, 118
  physical activity and, 116
  physician's role in, 123-124
  physiological factors in, 124
  psychological aspects of, 114-116
  psychological concomitants of infarction and, 114
  psychosocial resources of patient and family and, 125
  resources in, 125-126
  risk factors and life-style considered in, 116
  sexual problems and, 118-120, 162-171
  spouses of patients and, 116-118
  stages of recovery and, 114-115
  success of, 158
  team approach to, 126
  trust of patient and, 116
  vocational, 131-146
    assessment in, 138-139
    definition of, 137
    motivational considerations and, 142
    problems in, 132-136
    services in, 136-145
    stress inventory for, 143-144
    successful, 135
Rehabilitation counselor, 145
Reinforcement-control, 175
  drug regimens and, 183-184
Relaxation techniques, 161
Research as source of conflict in coronary care unit, 99
Reserpine, 168
Response, style of, and type A and type B behaviors, 18-19
Reticular activating system, 56
Risk factor(s)
  for angina pectoris, 6-7
  behavior patterns as, 7-14
  competitiveness and, 13
  for coronary disease
    biomedical, 51, 60
      control of, 59
    coronary-prone behavior pattern as, 24-25
    identification of, 85-86
    perceptual style and, 58
    psychosocial, 26
    reduction of
      behavioral approaches to, 172-189

Risk factor(s)—cont'd
reduction of—cont'd
educational approaches to, 173-174
role of individual differences in, 57-59
type A behavior and, 25
life-style and, 116
multiple, reduction of, 186-187
for myocardial infarction, 6-7
recurrent, type A behavior and, 23
striving for achievement as, 13
type A behavior as, studies in, 7-10
vocational involvement and, 12; *see also* Work

S

Scapegoating in coronary care unit, 98, 102, 103-104
Scheduling and staffing in coronary care unit, 99
Security of coronary patients, and nursing competence, 91
Sedation; *see* Medication(s)
Self-control, 175-176
Self-esteem
coronary care unit nurses and, 101, 109
myocardial infarction and, 93
Self-treatment and nontherapeutic activities, 72-74
Sensory information processing as determinant of cardiovascular function, 58
Sensory intake behavior, 53, 61
Sensory rejection behavior, 53-54
Serum cholesterol levels, 59
Sex
coronary disease and, 14
of patient and delay in seeking medical help, 69
Sexual activity
cardiovascular response to, 119
demands of, 119
effect of medications on, 120
fear of, 100-101
after myocardial infarction, 118-120, 133, 157
problems with, 119-120
Sexual counseling of coronary patients, 162-171
assessment and, 167-169
desire, decreased, and, 163
goal of, 166-167
inadequate, 166
sexual dysfunctions and, 162-163
factors in, 163-166
psychogenic, 170
therapy and, 170
Sexual misbehavior, 100-101
Sixteen Personality Factor Test, 7
Sleep disturbances
after myocardial infarction, 113
in rehabilitation, 114-115
Smoking cessation
aversive procedures for, 176-177
broad-spectrum programs for, 176, 178
environmental control and, 177-178
maintenance of, 178
skill training and, 177
social influence and, 178
Social Readjustment Rating Scale, 36-38
Speech hurrying, 18
Spouse(s) of coronary patients, 116-118; *see also* Family(ies) of coronary patients
distress and, 118
effect of myocardial infarction on, 113-114
family therapy and, 156-157
guilt and, 118
outpatient groups and, 118
oversolicitousness by, 117
sexual problems and, 118-120, 167
Stimulus-control, 175
drug regimens and, 183-184
Stress; *see also* Behavior(s); Conflict; Coping; specific issues
blood pressure elevations in response to, 52
cardiac output and, 55
cardiovascular response to, 56
of caring for terminal patients, 105-108
circle of, 180-181
coronary care unit experience and, 152-153
psychological intervention and, 153-158
coronary care unit nurses and, 101-103
group meetings for, 99-101
sources of, 101-103
coronary disease and, role of individual differences in, 57-59
defense reactions and, 56
definition of, 54-55
effect of, on synthesis of neurotransmitters, 57
hemodynamic responses to, 55
vascular beds and, 53
lipid metabolism levels and, 54
management of, training in, 181
occupational; *see* Work
psychosocial, effects of, on cardiovascular function, 57
reactions in, and coping behavior, 55
rehabilitation as source of, 159
serum cholesterol levels and, 59
skeletal muscle blood flow and, 54-55
sources of, 152, 159

Stress—cont'd
terminal patients, care of, and, 99
type A behavior and, 6
unnecessary, subsequent to myocardial infarction, 113
Success ethic, 12
Suicide, 158
Support for patient's personal needs, 157-158
Sympathetic nervous system
cardiovascular function and, 57, 61
function of, and perceptual styles, 59
increased activity of, and stress, 57
neurotransmitter synthesis in, and stress, 57
Symptom(s)
faulty attribution of, 68-69
onset of
day of, and decision time, 73
social context of, 71-72
time of day of, and decision time, 72
patient perception of, and preadmission behavior, 70-71
prodromal and delay in seeking medical help, 71

T

Teaching, patient
coronary care unit nurses and, 93-96
as means of psychological intervention, 153-154
spouses of coronary patients and, 118
Team approach to rehabilitation, 126, 142, 145
Terminal patient(s)
care of, 105-108
family of, 108
nurse-physician communication and, 106-107
staff conflict and, 106-107
stress involved in care of, 99
Thought, style of, type A and type B behaviors and, 16
Thousand Aviator Study, 59
Tranquilizers, 156
for cessation of smoking, 177
Transportation time, 68
Trappist-Benedictine Monastery study, 24
Treatment plans for terminal patients, 105-106
Tricyclic antidepressants, 156, 160
Twins and coronary death, 41
Type A behavior(s); *see also* Coronary-prone behavior pattern; Type A individual(s)
age and, 24-25
as all-or-none phenomenon, 24
atherosclerosis and, 8
behavior modification and, 180-182
characteristics of, 14-22
Type A behavior(s)—cont'd
clinical recognition of, 14-22
in coronary care unit, 22-24
coronary disease and, role of individual differences in, 57-59
depression and, susceptibility to, 159; *see also* Depression
description of, 6
distribution of
in United States population, 24
in Western Collaborative Group Study, 24
explanation of, to patient, 22-23
incidence of clinical coronary disease and, 8
intensity of, 25
Jenkins Activity Survey studies of, 8-10
life events and, 44-45
manifestations of, 14
occupational achievement and, 13; *see also* Work
operant approaches to modifications of, 181-182
population groups and, 24-25
as predictor of clinical subtypes of coronary disease, 25
questions about, 24-26
as risk factor for coronary disease, 7-14
across age groups and populations, 24-25
recurrent myocardial infarction and, 23
Western Collaborative Group Study findings and, 7-8, 9
socioeconomic status and, 24
stress and, 6
Type A individual(s); *see also* Coronary-prone personality; Type A behavior(s)
behavior of, 14-22
breathing of, 20-22
coronary atherosclerosis and, 50
facial expressions of, 19-20
gestures and movements of, 19
hostility by, 13-14
interpersonal relationships of, 16-18
involvement of family in rehabilitation of, 23-24
medical care of, 22-24
perceptual style of, 59
response style of, 18-19
serum cholesterol levels in, 59
therapeutic goals for, 23; *see also* Rehabilitation
thought style of, 16
values of, 15-16
women as, 24-25

Type B behavior(s); *see also* Type B individual(s)
  characteristics of, 14-22
  definition of, 6
  distribution of
    in United States population, 24
    in Western Collaborative Group Study, 24
  life events and, 45
  manifestations of, 14
Type B individual(s); *see also* Type B behavior(s)
  breathing of, 20-22
  facial expressions of, 19-20
  gestures and movements of, 19
  interpersonal relationships of, 16-18
  response style of, 18-19
  thought style of, 16
  values of, 15-16

V

Values, personal, type A and type B behaviors and, 15-16
Vascular resistance, forearm, and sensory intake behavior, 53-54
Vasoconstriction
  renal, stress and, 55
  in skeletal muscle during sensory intake behavior, 53, 54
Vasodilation and sensory rejection behavior, 53-54
Ventromedial nucleus; *see* Hypothalamus
Veterans Administration Collaborative Study, 51
Vocational rehabilitation; *see* Rehabilitation, vocational
Vocational tasks, 140
Voodoo death, 32

W

WCGS; *see* Western Collaborative Group Study
Weakness
  deconditioning and, 125
  depression and, 159; *see also* Depression
  after myocardial infarction, 113
  rehabilitation and, 114-115; *see also* Physical activity; Rehabilitation
Western Collaborative Group Study, 7-8
  distribution of type A and type B individuals in, 21
  methods of, 7
Women, postcoronary, and sexual disorders, 163
Work
  addiction to, 12
  problems in rehabilitation and, 123, 125
  reluctance of patient to return to, 113
  return to patient's health perception and, 113, 131-134, 136
    self-esteem and, 135
  satisfaction with, and coronary care unit nurses, 109-110

X

Xylocaine, 79